The Emotional Journey of the Alzheimer's Family

DARTMOUTH COLLEGE PRESS

HANOVER, NEW HAMPSHIRE

The Emotional Journey of the Alzheimer's Family

ROBERT B. SANTULLI, MD

KESSTAN BLANDIN, PHD

Dartmouth College Press
An imprint of University Press of New England
www.upne.com

Manufactured in the United States of America
Designed by Eric M. Brooks
Typeset in Calluna by Passumpsic Publishing

Library of Congress Cataloging-in-Publication Data
Santulli, Robert B.
The emotional journey of the Alzheimer's family / Robert B. Santulli, M.D., Kesstan Blandin, Ph.D.
pages cm
Includes bibliographical references and index.
ISBN 978-1-61168-773-6 (cloth : alk. paper)—
ISBN 978-1-61168-744-6 (pbk. : alk. paper)—
ISBN 978-1-61168-745-3 (ebook)
1. Alzheimer's disease—Patients—Family relationships. 2. Alzheimer's disease—Patients—Care. 3. Caregivers—Psychology.
I. Blandin, Kesstan. II. Title.
RC523.S277 2015
616.8'31—dc23 2014036572

Contents

Acknowledgments

Without a family, man, alone in the world,
trembles with the cold.
ANDRÉ MAUROIS

We wish to thank the many Alzheimer's families we have come to know and to care about deeply. They have permitted us to describe aspects of their lives here, in order to illuminate the points made in our writing. In all cases, we have changed names and altered identifying features in order to maintain anonymity, but we have attempted at the same time to clearly and accurately describe their struggles so that our words would not be merely dry and theoretical, but brought to life by the real experiences of our patients and their families. In many cases, these are people whom we have treated clinically. In some cases, they are individuals who have attended one of our support groups, educational sessions, or our Memory Café (Santulli 2013). They are the backbone of this volume in every way.

As we began our work on this book, Rocco D'Eugenio, one of our close relatives, began to show increasing signs of Alzheimer's disease, and he came to live in a local assisted living facility in order to be near us. Our relationship with this delightful man over the years of his illness until his death some months ago has been extremely poignant. He has taught us more about the emotional journey of the Alzheimer's family than we have learned in years of clinical work. We are deeply grateful for all that Rocco gave us, both when he was well and when he was ill. We miss him very much, indeed.

We would like to thank Alison Guh for the fine painting that has become the cover of this book. After learning what our work was about, she was able to capture the essence of the vital family relationships very effectively and artistically.

We wish to thank our wonderful editor, Phyllis Deutsch, editor in chief of the University Press of New England. Phyllis has had to endure us for much too long as we tried to write this manuscript, despite being much too busy with our other tasks. As a result, we too often proceeded at a snail's pace. Phyllis has been unfailingly kind and extraordinarily helpful with her comments, critiques, and suggestions as we have inched along. She has the patience of a saint.

We would also like to express our appreciation to Mary McLaughlin, writer and blogger, for permitting us to reprint her beautiful post about her father, "Zen and the Art of Alzheimer's" (McLaughlin 2013).

Writing a book with another person is a unique and very gratifying partnership. Our work with each other began with numerous discussions over lunch or coffee, and a mutual affection and respect for the other, personally and professionally. Those feelings have only grown as our work on the book proceeded to its conclusion. We would like to thank each other for the assistance, inspiration, patience, and friendship that each of us has given the other during this project.

Finally, our interest in writing about the Alzheimer's *family* grows directly from our deep connections to our own families and our awareness that there is nothing in life as important as family for comfort, support, help, reassurance, and love as we make our way on our own journeys. We are deeply, deeply grateful to our families.

The Emotional Journey of the Alzheimer's Family

Introduction

The Importance of Understanding the Family's Emotional and Psychological Experiences

In the United States today, nearly five and a half million individuals suffer from Alzheimer's disease, a chronic, progressive illness that affects memory, functioning, mood, personality, and behavior (Alzheimer's Association 2014). While there is much research being conducted to determine the cause or causes of Alzheimer's disease and to develop treatments more effective than those currently available, there is, at present, no way to prevent the condition, and there is no cure. Once someone has Alzheimer's disease, it will gradually worsen until death. Because of the aging of the population, if by the middle of this century no cure or prevention is developed, there may be as many as 15 million sufferers in the United States (Alzheimer's Association 2014). Alzheimer's disease is an epidemic rapidly reaching crisis proportions.

Much has been written for, or about, the primary caregiver, or to use the term preferred here, care partner. *Care partner* more accurately captures the complex and reciprocal relationship between the family member and the person with the disease. It is, indeed, a mutual partnership, rather than a relationship that is all "give" and no "take," although it might not always seem that way to overburdened care partners. While there usually is a *primary* care partner (often a spouse, if there is one), there are almost always several others who are directly involved, and deeply anguished, by the change in the person from a fully functioning, autonomous person to someone profoundly transformed by the ravages of the illness. Those affected include immediate family members living in the same household or nearby, as well as those family members who are geographically removed from the person with the disease but still quite attached and concerned. It also includes friends, close neighbors, and others whose lives are touched in some way by the person with the disease. It is this larger group that is signified by the term *Alzheimer's family* (Santulli 2011), and it is for this larger group that this book has been written. Its purpose is to consider the many ways in which the disease psychologically and emotionally affects the Alzheimer's family, in order to develop a deeper understanding of the deep anguish caused by losing a loved one to Alzheimer's. We trust that this will also lead to an enhanced ability to adapt to the changed individual and to the enormous burdens of having the disease in one's life. Finally, we hope that this examination of the emotional journey of the Alzheimer's family will help the affected family members achieve a greater degree of acceptance of this very challenging situation.

Much of what is written here applies to family members of persons with other types of dementia, as well. From the family's perspective, in particular, there are many similarities between the various types of dementia. This volume should therefore also be quite relevant to those who are family members of persons with non-Alzheimer's dementias.

Although there appears to be a significant preponderance of females with the illness (Alzheimer's Association 2014), Alzheimer's victims and Alzheimer's care partners obviously can be either male or female. So throughout this book, the awkward phrases "he or she," "his or her," "himself or herself," and the like, have been avoided, and one or the other gender is used, arbitrarily.

While all chronic, serious illnesses profoundly affect the victim's family members, it would seem that the impact of Alzheimer's disease on the family is particularly powerful and unique in its characteristics. It is often said that the burdens of this disease fall with even greater weight on the affected family members, compared with the victim himself. It is impossible, of course, to determine who suffers more — the person with the disease or the family. But it is very clear that the loads placed on both are enormous, and the suffering of the family adds immeasurably to the overall misery caused by this illness.

When family members are able to recognize, discuss, and successfully process the difficult feelings they experience, important benefits follow — both for the family and for the person with Alzheimer's. Gaining insight and understanding will make these powerful emotions seem less overwhelming and less controlling of the family members' daily lives. It will permit them to feel less victimized by the experience, more able to choose methods of coping with it, and thus better able to adapt to the situation. This will keep families healthier, both emotionally and physically, and more able to successfully meet the enormous demands of caring for the person with the illness. Family members will have more energy to devote to the many tasks involved and will be able to make better, more positive decisions regarding the person with Alzheimer's. They will react to the person with the disease with less anger, guilt, or other troubling and destructive feelings, and will be less likely to reach the dangerous endpoint of *care partner burnout*. All of this may lead to the family's being able to delay institutional placement by being better able to cope with the situation at home, or it may enable the family to make a more objective, thoughtful decision about placement, with less guilt, when that time comes. In addition, understanding and working through these feelings will free up significant amounts of emotional energy, permitting family members to lead more active and gratifying lives outside of the role of care partner, both during the illness and after.

It should be emphasized that the conceptualizations presented in this volume are exclusively those of the authors. They are drawn from more than thirty years' clinical experience caring for those with Alzheimer's disease and their family members. While not derived from evidenced-based literature, the ideas presented are consistent with research in these areas.

Challenges on the Journey

The emotional journey of the Alzheimer's family varies greatly from one household to the next. But there are a number of important challenges that most family care partners will encounter along the way. How each of these challenges is met will have an important impact on the next challenge that arises and on the journey as a whole.

Often, one of the earliest trials that occurs is a significant degree of *discordance* between the views of the disease held by the person with Alzheimer's, on the one hand, and those of the family, on the other. Typically, the person with the disease has less awareness of her symptoms than the family, and she may be quite vigorous in her denial of the problem. This can create significant tension between the family and the person with the illness; it can also lead to a delay in diagnosis, poor compliance with treatment, and a reluctance or unwillingness to accept measures that are necessary to maintain safety. While this discordance generally first presents itself early in the course of illness, it can continue in various forms throughout the disease. Discordance is a major source of emotional stress and burden for the Alzheimer's family. Factors that contribute to discordance are reviewed, the implications of significant discordance are discussed, and methods to diminish it are considered in chapter 2. Another common issue is the use of various *defenses* by family members to avoid or lessen the impact of the reality of the patient's disease and all the implications associated with it. The use of defenses by family members is also addressed in chapter 2.

In the course of coping with the illness in a loved one, family members commonly experiences a number of strong emotions: these include anger, guilt, anxiety, shame, and, of course, grief.

While grief is at the center of every family member's emotional experience, not every family member experiences each of the other four emotions with equal intensity. At times, these other emotions can also serve a defensive purpose: being preoccupied with anger, guilt, anxiety, or shame may prevent the family member from facing the even greater anguish of grief. Anxiety, guilt, anger, and shame are discussed in chapter 3.

Grief, the central emotional response to losing a loved one, before physical death occurs, is introduced in chapter 4. This chapter brings clarity to those aspects of grief that are unique to Alzheimer's disease, owing not only to the sheer number of significant losses suffered but also to the specific nature of these losses.

Family care partners who have experienced the grief of having a loved one with Alzheimer's disease must go through a difficult process of *adaptation*, in order to move forward, while remaining emotionally connected and available to their loved one who has been transformed by this disease. This important topic is considered in chapter 5.

Of course, family members do not experience the various psychological and emotional elements of this journey in a neat, orderly fashion. It might be tempting to imagine, for example, that once discordance and defenses are overcome, the family member will next move on to the common emotional reactions mentioned above, deal with these, and then proceed to work through the core feelings of grief. Unfortunately, the situation is much more complex than that, and it may even seem chaotic at times. Emotions, defenses, and discordances happen in any order, or all at the same time. While the family member is struggling with her own feelings about the disease, she may also be utilizing a variety of defenses to lessen their emotional impact, while at the same time she is attempting to address the discordance between herself and the person with the disease regarding their differing views of the illness. Emotions, defenses, and discordances come and go in various combinations and with differing intensities throughout the disease, depending on external events, the specific characteristics of illness, and the particular personalities of the family member and the person with the disease.

One implication of this fact is that the family member faces a very complex psychological and emotional challenge in trying to cope with a loved one with Alzheimer's disease. A second implication is that the family member cannot, unfortunately, address one element, finish with it, and go on to the next. Different phases of the illness, the appearance of new symptoms or new impairments, or changes in life circumstances can bring forth new discordances, new defenses, and new emotional responses. It is only by repeatedly wrestling with the different components of this emotional and psychological web that the family member can ultimately master her anguish and begin to adapt in a positive and healthy fashion to the losses brought about by the disease.

Beyond Grief to Acceptance

Chapter 6, "Acceptance and Moving Forward," focuses on how Alzheimer's family members can progress from grief to a state of equanimity, acceptance, and personal growth. Having experienced deep feelings of grief, how does the Alzheimer's family member come to terms with the illness in her loved one? How does she reach a degree of *acceptance*, not just feeling emotionally exhausted and saddened, but also enhanced and affirmed—bettered, even? Some features in the relationship between the person with Alzheimer's and the family member that are associated with positive outcomes are reviewed, and some of the individual personality characteristics of the family member that are especially valuable in coping with this journey in a healthy and constructive fashion are presented. Finally, some of the families discussed earlier in the book will be revisited, to examine how they reached—or didn't reach—this final stage of acceptance.

Although much of the effort of coming to terms with losing a loved one to Alzheimer's disease is internal and psychological, there are important interpersonal and social dimensions to the healing process, as well. In chapter 7, some very specific ways in which the Alzheimer's family can connect to the Alzheimer's community to form vital bonds with other care partners and families are discussed. Because of the stigma surrounding Alzheimer's disease, this can be a challenging task, but it is a very necessary one. Connecting with the Alzheimer's community is a crucial tool in adaptation and in moving beyond the sense of grief at the core of losing a loved one to this illness.

Chapter 8 reviews the causes and features of the care partner's burden. Some of the risks that these problems pose to both the care partner and the person with the illness are considered. This final chapter also presents a number of important tenets that every family care partner should consider in order to lessen the degree of their troubles, and to cope more effectively with the inevitable stress that is present. The varieties of professional help that are available for the severely stressed care partner are also reviewed.

Chapter One
Coping with Discordant Views of the Illness

In the majority of people with Alzheimer's disease, the individual with the disease is less aware of the illness, its severity, and its consequences than are members of the family. While there are exceptions to this pattern, there is commonly a significant discordance between the person with the disease and the family member regarding the presence or extent of Alzheimer's disease. The gulf that so often exists between the family's view, on the one hand, and the view of the person with the disease, on the other, is one of the most distressing and difficult aspects of the family's attempt to cope with the illness, particularly in the early stages.

Factors Leading to Discordance

Several elements contribute to this discordance. One is simply the memory impairment itself, which is, of course, a hallmark of the disease. The person with Alzheimer's often cannot *recall* previous events related to cognitive difficulties. As family members will often say, "he forgets that he forgets."

Patricia had been suffering from Alzheimer's disease for about five years. She had very poor recent memory and difficulty naming her four children or knowing much about their current lives (marriages, careers, and so forth), even though all lived in the area and visited regularly. From time to time, she would ask for her mother, who had been dead for several decades.

Patricia had not worked outside the home since her children

were born. She had been a good housekeeper, managing the children's busy school and activity schedules with ease and with enjoyment when they were young.

Over the past year or more, Patricia pursued very few activities. She refused to go to the local senior center and spent much of the day in front of the television or napping. However, when asked what she did with her time, she would state without hesitation that she spent the day doing housekeeping, including dusting, vacuuming, laundry, and making dinner for her husband, Ted, every night. In reality, she had done none of the housekeeping for the past year at least, other than to occasionally help Ted fold the laundry, and sometimes she would cut vegetables for their dinner salad, under Ted's close supervision.

On one occasion, after hearing her outline her supposed activities on a typical day, Ted asked her what type of vacuum cleaner they had. She described an upright version with a long handle. In fact, the vacuum she described may have been one they had many years ago; they now owned a round one that rolled around on the floor, not an upright model. It seemed likely that in describing her typical day, Pat was recalling her activities (and her vacuum cleaner) from many years ago, believing that she was talking about the present, as is so often the case in persons with Alzheimer's disease. Certainly, she was not consciously telling lies about her current activity; she genuinely believed that what she recalled doing in the more remote past was what she was doing at the present time.

....

A second factor contributing to discordance is the use of the defense of *denial* by the person with Alzheimer's disease (Ogden and Biebers 2010). This is a common defense mechanism used by all persons, to some degree. Denial is a psychological process that involves the active rejection from consciousness of a painful or frightening reality. People with Alzheimer's commonly use denial to avoid some of the more emotionally painful and frightening elements of the disease. So do their family members. Denial, as well as other defense mechanisms used by family members is presented in the next chapter. The discordance in the views between the person with Alzheimer's and the family is often attributed to denial, exclusively, but the process is more complex, including forgetfulness and several other factors, described below.

A third factor that leads to discordance between how the family and the afflicted individual view the illness is a phenomenon known as *anosognosia* (Starkstein et al. 2006). Anosognosia is a neurological term that refers to the inability to recognize deficits, because of some form of brain damage. Anosognosia can occur in a variety of neurological and psychiatric conditions, such as stroke or schizophrenia, in addition to Alzheimer's disease. Some use the term *unawareness* as a synonym for anosognosia.

....

Martin, a sixty-seven-year-old man who did *not* have Alzheimer's disease, suffered a stroke in the right temporoparietal area of his brain. As a result, he lost not only the ability to move his left arm, but also lost his ability to *recognize* the deficit. While still recovering in the hospital, his wife would attempt to get him to exercise the afflicted arm, but he would refuse to do so. When asked why, he explained his paralysis by stating that his arm was just very tired, and he did not feel like moving it. On other occasions, when asked to move his left arm, he moved his right arm instead but stated (and seemed to believe) that he was moving his left one.

....

This was not conscious deception on Martin's part, and it is not conscious fabrication when a similar phenomenon occurs related to cognition in the person with Alzheimer's. The ability to recognize the impairment has been lost, owing to brain damage. In the case of the person with Alzheimer's, it can be quite difficult to tell whether the lack of awareness is psychologically motivated—that is, resulting from denial—or is neurologically caused (anosognosia), or if it has simply been forgotten (a recent memory deficit). For example, the person with Alzheimer's who states that she has a very good memory when that is clearly no longer the case may be suffering from denial, or this could represent anosognosia. It could also be simple forgetting. In any case, it is good for the family to keep anosognosia in mind when the person with the disease does not recognize her deficits.

A fourth factor that contributes to the discordance of views is the *stigma* that is frequently felt about Alzheimer's disease and the consequent fear of social disapproval that is often experienced by its victims (Jolley and Benbow 2000). Unfortunately, this continues, despite the important improvements in care developed over the past decades, and despite the fact that increasing numbers of prominent figures, beginning with Ronald Reagan, have publicly discussed their own Alzheimer's disease.

The Origins of Alzheimer's Stigma

From childhood, students are taught that to remember well is a valued ability. A great deal of learning in school—particularly for earlier generations—has been based on rote memorization and the ability to recall. When students remember very well, they get good grades on tests, win the praise of their teachers and parents, are placed in advanced classes, get into good colleges, and the like. On the other hand, those who don't remember well do poorly on exams and are often thought of as "stupid" or "lazy." Thus, from childhood, poor remembering (whether because of inherent lack of ability or effort) is viewed negatively, and those who are poor at remembering, for whatever reason, are socially devalued, or stigmatized. Later in life, the ability to learn quickly and to remember remains a valued trait. The salesman who excels at remembering his customers' names and personal attributes, or the employee who is able to learn a new routine quickly and well in the factory or in the office will advance, whereas those who have trouble mastering these tasks tend to fall behind or fail.

While today's educational system may be moving away from the focus on rote memorization, placing more emphasis on understanding concepts and other factors, one's ability to learn and remember well remain highly valued abilities that are associated with success in school, and the opposite is linked with poor performance or failure and is highly stigmatized. This value system continues throughout life and carries into old age. It is a part of the reason why those who remember especially poorly—those with Alzheimer's disease—often meet with social disapproval or stigmatization and why a common response of care partners and others to someone who is beginning to forget is to encourage them to "try harder"—as if a greater effort, just as in school, will solve the problem.

In the case of Alzheimer's disease, there are other factors, as well, that contribute to the sense of stigmatization, in addition to forgetfulness. Society places great emphasis on the ability to control one's public behavior, to appear and act appropriately in all situations. Unfortunately, people with Alzheimer's gradually lose this ability in the course of the disease. As a result, they may say or do odd things, appear unkempt or disheveled, speak when or where it is inappropriate to do so, yell or curse in public, use poor manners at the table, and the like. While none of these behaviors should be viewed as the "fault" of the person with the disease, nevertheless, this loss of control of one's behaviors tends to be viewed negatively by others. This is another factor that contributes to the stigmatization of those with the disease.

Frequently, the sense of stigma extends as well to the care partner, who may be "painted with the same brush." This has been labeled as "stigma by association," or "courtesy stigma" (Werner and Heinik 2008). In addition to prejudice that the family care partner experiences from others regarding the loved one's dementia, she may also hold certain prejudicial or stigmatic beliefs *herself* regarding the illness. This can certainly contribute to the defenses used and emotions experienced by the care partner. These issues are discussed in more detail in the following chapters. Positive ways of coping with stigma are discussed in chapter 7, "Connecting with the Alzheimer's Community."

Of course, not everyone views Alzheimer's disease, and those who suffer from it, in this devalued manner. Many, particularly those who have a family member with the disease, are quite understanding and sympathetic. However, others may simply be terrified of the disease and its victims. Alzheimer's is the most feared illness among the elderly (Marist Institute for Public Opinion 2012), and a frequent method of dealing with fear is *avoidance*. Many people with Alzheimer's disease, and sometimes even their care partners, are shunned for this reason. People with the disease may be avoided by others because they are devalued, seen as socially unacceptable, or simply because others want to avoid being confronted with the reality that they could easily be in the same situation, themselves. The result of this avoidance for those with Alzheimer's, and to some extent for their family members, is isolation and stigmatization.

Although the person with Alzheimer's disease may not be able to verbalize about feeling stigmatized—a concept, however real, that is nevertheless too abstract for many with the disease—individuals with Alzheimer's, especially early in the disease process, are frequently all too aware that aspects of their functioning and behavior meet with disapproval from those around them, and they may well feel further diminished by these negative attributions. This helps explain why people with the disease automatically try to hide their cognitive difficulties from others as much as possible, at least while the ability to do so still exists.

Whether the problem is due to anosognosia, denial, forgetting, stigma, or the fear of social disapproval, or some combination of all of these, the lack of recognition of deficits is generally not conscious or volitional on the part of the person with the impairment, although it can certainly seem as if it is. Reminding oneself of the involuntary nature of this behavior caused by the disease can help lessen the frustration or anger that family members may experience otherwise.

The concept of discordance includes all of the components mentioned above, to a varying degree. It also emphasizes the interpersonal nature of this phenomenon, by including in its definition not only on the person with the disease, but also the family care partner. The implication of discordance is that there is a difference of opinion between the disease victim and the family member, and it is this discrepancy that creates tension for the family care partner. Occasionally, a situation occurs in which the person with the disease is in total denial of his illness, and the care partner is equally in denial of the illness. Although this is uncommon, and often doesn't last very long, in such a situation there is *no* discordance. Both individuals view the disease in the same, albeit distorted, fashion.

Family Reactions to Discordant Views about the Disease

How do family members typically respond to the person with Alzheimer's who does not see her illness realistically? Some family members might argue with the person, insisting that she does indeed have a problem and that she needs to recognize and accept it. This approach is rarely helpful. The person with the disease will likely become more defensive, and often both parties end up feeling angry. Simple insistence does not reduce denial.

On the other hand, the complete avoidance of talking about this discordance creates a widening gulf between the family member and the person with the disease. Particularly when the family member is a spouse, there probably has never been an issue in their relationship that has been so fundamentally important—and where opinions are so fundamentally in disagreement. This disagreement is often greater than any differences the couple may have had about other basic subjects, such as religion, politics, or sex. The emotional strain caused by this discordance is a major source of stress and unhappiness for family members. Both the family member and the person with the disease can understandably become quite upset by the tension and arguing that discordance creates.

Family members who avoid any discussion of this discordance usually give several reasons for this. Understandably, they do not wish to cause conflict with the loved one and worry that if they bring up the issue, it is likely to lead to defensiveness and arguing, or worse. In addition, they do not want to raise an issue that they feel will diminish her dignity. And they certainly do not wish to cause her distress, as they are quite aware that living with the disease is already quite frustrating and painful for the disease victim.

In addition, some family members believe that telling the person with the disease that she has Alzheimer's will cause harm. The family may fear that she will become so despondent over the news that she will give up trying to function or will become suicidal. However, studies that have examined the effect of disclosing the diagnosis have not found any harmful effect from this, even if it is upsetting initially (Carpenter et al. 2008).

Many people with Alzheimer's disease will, from time to time, make a statement about wanting life to be over. This is generally caused by the awareness of and frustration over difficulties with remembering and functioning, and it usually does not represent an active desire to end one's life. In general, the more families talk about the disease, by name, the *less* likely it is that the person with Alzheimer's will feel the desire to end her life. The sense of connection to the family is probably the strongest factor that protects against the desire for suicide, and being able to openly discuss what is wrong certainly reinforces that sense of connection. In any case, it is extremely rare that individuals with the disease actually attempt self-harm. And if they do, there is no relationship to whether or not they have been told they have Alzheimer's disease.

In fact, the person with Alzheimer's disease often becomes less upset with the diagnosis than family members do. This may be because the person with the disease suspects it, or because he has already lost the ability to be concerned about the full implications of having this illness. Nevertheless, families often assume that the news will devastate the person with the disease, as it has devastated them, but this is usually not the case. It is important to remember that it is the disease that is devastating, and not simply its label. However, for all of the reasons outlined above, there often exists a "conspiracy of silence" in which both the person with the disease and the family member are very aware that something is wrong, but neither wants to bring it up for fear of upsetting the other.

....

Mark and Joanna went for Mark's initial memory clinic evaluation accompanied by their daughters, Abigail and Bridget. Joanna had initiated the evaluation because of her concerns about Mark's increasing forgetfulness. However, she said to Mark that the evaluation was for the purpose of checking his stress levels, since he seemed more "tense" recently. Mark viewed the questionnaire that had been sent to Joanna to complete prior to the appointment and easily surmised that the real reason for the evaluation was his growing cognitive difficulties. However, he never mentioned to her that he had seen the questionnaire prior to the appointment. Shortly before his scheduled clinic visit, the physician received a telephone call from Joanna. She asked that "if he has Alzheimer's, don't tell him—it will kill him." On the day of the appointment, the doctor greeted the family in the waiting room and asked them to follow him to the office. On the walk from the waiting room to the office, Mark pulled the doctor aside and whispered, "If I have Alzheimer's, don't tell my family—they'll be devastated."

Toward the end of the evaluation, one of Mark's daughters directly asked the doctor if Mark had Alzheimer's disease. The physician hesitated to respond, based on the clear messages that both Mark and Joanna had given. He indicated that he felt it was best to discuss the diagnosis openly, if all agreed. They did, at this point. They were told that the likely diagnosis was, in fact, mild Alzheimer's disease. Certainly, no one was glad to hear this, but it was clear that no one was surprised, either. Importantly, no one appeared to be devastated by the diagnosis. Mark and Joanna had never used the word Alzheimer's in discussing Mark's forgetfulness, and they were strongly encouraged to do so from this point forward. This marked the beginning of a greater degree of openness between Mark and Joanna concerning his illness.

....

Telling someone explicitly that she has Alzheimer's doesn't make the disease worse or better, of course, but it does permit people to talk about it openly. Maintaining a "conspiracy of silence" or facade that nothing is wrong, when in reality the lives of the person with the disease and the family have been fundamentally changed, wastes a great deal of energy on the part of both participants. This is energy that would be better spent dealing openly with the disease. Facing this "elephant in the room" can certainly be difficult at first, but people who have broken through the barrier of silence and have begun to speak frankly with their loved ones about Alzheimer's usually feel a great sense of relief, and an enhanced sense of closeness. They find that the overall burdens of the disease are much more manageable when everything is out in the open.

Often, however, family members feel that they do not know how to bring up the subject in a constructive fashion or in a way that will not anger, upset, or diminish the dignity of the person with the disease. So they say nothing—at least until some symptom or other stressful disease-related event makes them angry, and then they may say something about it in a less than optimal or sympathetic way. It would seem that the majority of people with Alzheimer's disease are quite aware, on some level, that something is wrong, even if they do not want to talk about it or if they do not fully understand the dimensions of the problem or its implications. For this reason, when a family member does bring up the subject with the person who has the disease, one reaction the person with the disease *rarely* shows is surprise. Among the most important tasks the family member must undertake, at this point, is to create opportunities to talk openly and dispassionately about the illness, so that this critical issue in their lives is not artificially kept out of open communication.

These discussions may be the most difficult in marital relationships that are distant or conflict-ridden in the first place. Similarly, when the family member is an adult child, talking about the illness openly is often the most problematic when the parent-child relationship is one characterized either by idealization of the parent, or when the adult child feels intimidated by, fearful of, or chronically angry at the parent with the disease. But these relationships—already conflicted in the first place—will only grow more distant if the subject continues to be avoided, and this puts increasing strain on the already-stressed family.

Lessening Discordance

Denial and the other factors contributing to discordance cannot be forcefully or suddenly eliminated by any action of the individual, the family member, or anyone else; to a great degree, the awareness and acceptance of the illness in the person with Alzheimer's disease will occur at its own pace. Indeed, there are some couples or families where the word *Alzheimer's* is never spoken, despite years of symptoms, and perhaps years of taking medications that are prescribed for Alzheimer's disease, as the person can learn from reading the package insert or from watching advertisements on television. In these families, there may be no discussion at all of cognitive difficulties, although continuing that subterfuge as the disease progresses becomes increasingly difficult and stressful. We do not believe that this approach is optimal, but we recognize that the dynamics of some families are such that some may see avoidance as the only way the matter can be handled. Before reaching that conclusion, however, it would be useful for the family to consider if avoidance is truly necessary for the benefit of the person with Alzheimer's, or whether it might be, in fact, the *family* that does not wish to face the issue themselves. In such a situation, it would be valuable to consult with an experienced clinician.

There are a number of approaches to dealing with this discordance. We believe that, very often, these approaches can help the person with Alzheimer's become more realistic about her illness and can make room for more open discussion of the situation sooner rather than later. First of all, it is important to realize that it is exceptionally difficult, if not impossible, to reduce denial or other sources of discordance in the person with Alzheimer's disease as long as members of the family are also in significant denial about the illness. Even when the majority of family members are realistic about the situation, if there is any involved family member who still has prominent denial, the person with Alzheimer's will sense the attitude of that person and will firmly align herself with that attitude.

....

Margaret was diagnosed with Alzheimer's disease about two years ago. She and her husband, Stephen, rarely talked about the illness, as doing so seemed to do little other than irritate Margaret and increase the general level of stress in the household. As the disease progressed, Stephen (who still worked full time) became increasingly concerned about leaving Margaret at home during the day. After a visit from the fire department because Margaret set off the smoke alarm by forgetting a pan on the stove, Stephen came to feel that he needed to have someone stay with Margaret while he was at work. Not wanting to impose this unilaterally, he asked her if she would mind having a companion while he was at work. Margaret firmly objected to the idea; she felt that she was perfectly fine to stay alone, and she minimized the kitchen incident. Stephen and their daughter, Emma, felt strongly that someone needed to be with Margaret so that she was not left alone at home. However, their son, Vincent, felt that perhaps his mother had just been careless in the kitchen, and if a note were placed on the stove to remind Margaret to turn off the burners after using them, this would be sufficient. Margaret most likely would have acquiesced to having someone at the house if the family had presented a single point of view, but after hearing Vincent's denial-based opinion, Margaret herself stood firmly against having someone stay at the house with her when Stephen was out, saying that if Vincent did not think it was necessary, then Stephen and Emma were wrong, and she would be fine staying home alone.

....

This example indicates the importance of the family presenting a unified opinion when discussing difficult issues such as these. If there is debate and lack of consensus about the issue among family members, it is best for everyone, particularly the person with Alzheimer's, to have this settled before the issue is raised with the person with the disease.

Family members often need to be convinced of the importance of discussing the disease openly with their loved one, and they need to feel confident that doing so will not harm the person with the disease, even if it is initially difficult and upsetting. Eventually, many family members will reach this opinion on their own, or with the help of a confidante, or perhaps through attending a support group. Once the family member recognizes the importance of talking to the loved one openly about the disease, he will usually be able to find ways to discuss the illness-related concerns with his loved one. In this regard, there are several principles that bear mentioning:

First, it is important to bring the subject up regularly, taking into account the fact that the person with Alzheimer's is likely to forget some or all of the conversations. There can be a fine line between being repetitive about an important topic, and badgering the person with the disease; certainly one wants to avoid the latter. Generally, it is best to bring it up when examples of forgetfulness or other cognitive symptoms have occurred, rather than at other times, and also to be careful to avoid anger and an attitude of "I told you so."

....

Tyler and his wife, Gertrude, have lived together happily for more than fifty years. Gradually, Tyler began to notice that Gertrude was becoming forgetful and, in particular, was constantly losing things around the house—keys, eyeglasses, purse, the portable telephone, for example. Tyler had become increasingly concerned about her behavior, and tried to discuss this with Gertrude, but Gertrude dismissed the incidents as "senior moments" that "happen to everyone" her age. Nevertheless, she was annoyed by having to spend so much time hunting for these essential items, and she usually asked Tyler to help her find them. The missing items always turned up but sometimes in unexpected and sometimes very peculiar locations. For example, after looking for Gertrude's wallet for more than a week, Tyler unexpectedly came upon it on their potting bench in the garage. Gertrude had no idea how it ended up there. Tyler decided that whenever Gertrude would lose something, he would help her look for it, as usual, and when it was eventually found, he would mention that he understood how frustrating it must be for her; but he would add that she should consider that the problem might be a sign of her having more memory trouble than she cared to recognize. In response, Gertrude blamed her losing things on having "senior moments" and on having too much clutter in the house. As Tyler persisted in gently bringing this up each time she lost something, she finally agreed, with some reluctance and a clear sense of humiliation, that this was a problem she should discuss with her doctor.

....

Some family members may feel that it is better to talk about the disease when everything is going "smoothly." While that reasoning is understandable and may work well for some, discussing the problems at such a time may, in fact, not be very successful. If episodes of forgetting or other symptoms have not just occurred, the person with the disease may simply not remember any of the problems she has had and will not be able to relate to the concerns the family member is raising. Whatever the best time for discussing this might be for a particular individual, the important concept is that the illness should become an open and permitted topic of regular family conversation, not something that is only talked about in times of crisis and avoided at other times.

Who should be involved in these discussions will differ in each family. Some will want to restrict this discussion to only the immediate family members, or only between husband and wife. Other families are comfortable sharing this with a wider group. People with Alzheimer's disease and their family members are best served by talking openly about the disease with those who have regular, personal contact with the disease victim. This may not be the case for some families, and each must decide, with the person with the disease, who should be informed, and in what detail. It is also important to determine whether the desire to keep the disease hidden is coming from the person with the disease or from the family members themselves. Much of the reluctance to discuss this is due to the stigma surrounding the disease, which only adds to the burden that people with Alzheimer's and their families feel.

Second, it is obvious that the illness needs to be discussed in a nonjudgmental fashion. Alzheimer's is not the fault of the person with the disease, and it is important for family members to work very hard to keep the afflicted individual from feeling blamed for her problems. Symptoms do not, of course, represent a personal shortcoming or moral failure, and the family's talking about the illness should not be viewed as insulting to or critical of the person with the disease, although it often is viewed that way by individuals who are very defensive about having memory problems. Even though the need to be nonjudgmental is self-evident, very difficult interactions can occur when a family member does harbor judgmental attitudes, perhaps unconsciously.

....

Howard and Melinda have been married for many decades, but it has not been an ideal relationship. Howard is extremely bright and was a very successful stockbroker before his retirement. Since retiring, he has been actively involved with the school board and other community activities. Melinda has always been quiet, struggling with feelings of inferiority throughout much of her life. She was used to being in Howard's shadow but took pride in her home and in her ability to entertain their friends and his business associates with grace. Howard had always been somewhat critical of her, and throughout their marriage she has vacillated from feeling she needed to improve in some way, to feeling intense resentment and anger toward him for his sense of superiority and somewhat condescending attitude toward her. More than once, she considered leaving him, but never did, feeling that she could not manage on her own.

Although Howard is five years older than Melinda, he is in excellent physical health and mentally very sharp. Melinda, however, gradually developed forgetfulness for recent events, and other cognitive signs of Alzheimer's disease. She was initially quite defensive about it, particularly when Howard would point out events she had forgotten or errors she had made. The tension between them grew significantly. Objectively, Melinda's symptoms were in the mild range of impairment, and with proper supports in place she could function reasonably well. However, Howard saw her, and described her to others, as severely impaired. It was clear from speaking with them both, individually and as a couple, that although Howard paid lip service to the notion that the illness was an unfortunate turn of events over which she had no control, in reality (and unconsciously) he felt otherwise: he seemed to view Melinda's illness as shameful, and something that she could counteract if only she tried hard enough. Although Howard insisted, and clearly believed, that he only pointed out Melissa's symptoms in an effort to be helpful to her, she found his comments about her illness to be insulting, seeing them as attacks that were unkind and unjustified, and she argued angrily with him whenever he raised the subject. In return, he viewed her angry rejoinders as more symptoms of the disease, further "proof" of his view of her.

....

The unfortunate situation between Howard and Melinda should make clear how difficult it is to discuss Alzheimer's disease when there is a lack of basic closeness and trust in the marital bond in the first place. It is not surprising that Alzheimer's disease, like most other adversities, is more easily borne in the context of an intimate and loving relationship, although it can certainly cause strain in even the strongest of marriages or families.

The third principle that will facilitate productive discussion about the illness is that whenever one brings up the symptoms, it is important to counterbalance this with a comment about the person's preserved abilities or valued characteristics that remain intact (Beatty et al. 1994). Most individuals with Alzheimer's disease experience the illness as a significant assault on their self-esteem, even if few are able to talk about that spontaneously, or openly. Too often, there is an excessive focus on what is going wrong, rather than on the considerable amount of the self that remains intact, even in the later stages of the disease. It is incumbent on the family member to take stock of the preserved capabilities and characteristics that remain, so that these can be emphasized to the individual in a way that is genuine, and not patronizing. Doing so can help maintain the self-esteem of the person with Alzheimer's disease. Doing so will also facilitate the lessening of denial sufficiently so that the illness can be discussed more openly between the victim and the family.

Chapter Two

The Defenses of the Alzheimer's Family Care Partner

The emotional realities that confront Alzheimer's family members can be grim and cause intense anguish. This involves nothing less than having to face the gradual loss of the loved one in nearly every respect, often long before actual physical death occurs. For the spouse, it means facing the loss of a companion, a friend, a confidante, and a lover. It usually means facing the loss of the person upon whom one relies for counsel, advice, and concrete help with numerous family and household tasks. It also forces the spouse to cope with the difficult transition from having a partner in a mutually caring relationship to having someone who has become extremely dependent and needs increasing amounts of supervision and care. For the adult child, many of these same changes occur; in addition, the adult child has to cope with the reversal of roles from being the child to becoming the parent in many respects. Other family members face similar painful emotions as they cope with the loss of their relative to this terrible disease. Although, as discussed in the previous chapter, family members typically see the disease more completely and more realistically than the disease victim, it is nevertheless understandable that any family member facing this situation would develop strategies for coping with its emotional realities, in order to blunt their intensity or to face them gradually rather than all at once. Family members employ psychological defense mechanisms for this purpose.

Defenses Defined

A defense mechanism can be thought of as a self-deception, or a reality-distortion—a mental "trick" one plays on oneself in an attempt to adapt to something that is unpleasant, distressing, frightening, or anxiety-provoking. These self-deceptions are not consciously invoked but instead seem to happen automatically, coming (as the Freudians would say) from the unconscious. One is generally not aware of acting "defensively" unless someone points it out, and then the individual often strongly resists acknowledging that it is true. Most people like to think that their mental functioning is based entirely on rational thinking and that they are able to see and analyze whatever occurs in a perfectly clear and objective way, without any "rose-colored" or other distorting lenses. Of course, many things—perhaps most—are handled that way. For example, if someone is getting ready to leave the house and it is raining, he will probably don a raincoat, or carry an umbrella—rational responses to weather. However, he might instead deal with the unpleasant reality of rain in other ways: by avoiding it, "sugar-coating" it, rationalizing it, or in some other manner not completely facing it, at least initially. This is especially true if there is some uncertainty or ambiguity about the situation, as is so often the case in Alzheimer's.

If it is not raining, but the sky is filled with dark clouds, and the forecast warns of a high chance of precipitation, he might react to this in several ways. He might feel disappointed because he was hoping for good weather, but grab a raincoat or take an umbrella with him as he heads out the door. On the other hand, he might take an approach that is less based on the realities of the situation and instead utilizes defense mechanisms. Thus, he might notice the threatening skies but then avoid checking the weather forecast on the radio, not wanting to hear that it will likely rain. This is the defense mechanism of "avoidance." Alternatively, he might listen to the weather forecast but then decide that it probably won't rain after all, since the meteorologist is often wrong. This is an example of "rationalization" at work. Another defensive response he might employ is to think that even if it does rain, he probably will not get too wet, because there are only a few blocks to walk to get to where he is going. This could be seen as the defense of "minimization."

He may feel less distressed about the weather before he leaves the house if he adopts one of these defensive attitudes, but this approach won't stop it from raining, certainly, and he is more likely to get wet than if he had been more realistic to begin with. This example illustrates that while defenses may have an immediate anxiety-lessening effect, they can sometimes lead to more difficulties than facing the situation openly without defenses in the first place. Having a loved one with Alzheimer's, of course, causes infinitely greater distress than that caused by a rainy day, and therefore the motivation to use defenses is correspondingly greater. But the principles are the same.

Specific Defense Mechanisms Used by the Alzheimer's Family Member

This review of the defenses commonly used by family members is by no means a comprehensive exposition on the psychology of defensive functioning. For a definitive discussion of this topic, the works of Anna Freud (1937) and George Vaillant (1992) are recommended. Discussed here are only those defenses that are most frequently utilized by the Alzheimer's family member in order to avoid, lessen, or delay the anguish caused by this terrible disease. A thorough understanding of these defenses will make it easier for the open-minded individual reading this volume to be able to identify patterns in her own ways of reacting. Ideally, this will lead to self-reflection and to candid discussions with family, friends, a health-care professional, or the members of a support group. Reflecting on one's own defensive behaviors and talking with concerned others will lead to an increase in insight and self-knowledge, as well as an enhanced ability to openly face the realities of the current circumstances. Ultimately, this will be helpful both to the family member and to the person with Alzheimer's disease.

The general principles of defensive mental operations are more important than the specific labels given to the various mechanisms to be described. At times, a particular behavior may represent an amalgam of more than one defense mechanism, or it could be described equally accurately by more than one label. Although each defense mechanism will be discussed by name, the more important issue is the general psychological process of trying to protect oneself from painful realities, and the cost exacted by doing so.

Repression

Repression involves the automatic excluding from one's mind an idea that is unpleasant, frightening, or anxiety-provoking. It is different from simply deciding not to think about something; that involves a conscious decision, whereas repression is automatic, taking place without any conscious awareness.

....

Mike and Helen had been married for forty-two years. Mike deeply loved Helen, who had early Alzheimer's disease. One day, Mike noticed that Helen had placed one of her shoes in the refrigerator. This was quite upsetting to Mike, and when he asked Helen about it, she was not able to offer any explanation. Mike mentioned it to his daughter, Erika, on the telephone later that day, still bothered by it. Two weeks later, at her regular medical checkup, Helen's physician asked Mike if there had been any unusual behaviors. Mike thought about the question and was only able to indicate that, at times, Helen asked repetitive questions. That night, when talking with his daughter on the phone about the appointment, Erika asked her father if he had told the doctor about the shoe in the refrigerator. Mike stated that he had not, that he had in fact completely forgotten about the incident that moment. Mike had no cognitive problems himself: this "forgetting" seemed instead to represent an example of repression at work. Putting her shoe in the refrigerator was a disturbing behavior of Helen's that Mike handled simply by pushing it out of his conscious mind.

Some time later, Helen complained that the television set was broken; she was unable to get it to change channels. When Mike explored the situation, it became apparent that the problem was that Helen was no longer able to operate the remote for the TV correctly. Mike carefully explained how to use the remote control device. A week or so later, when Erika was visiting, she noted that her mother was unable to work the television remote. Mike initially felt some surprise at this; it was only when he looked again at the TV and the remote (wanting to make sure it wasn't broken) that he recalled the previous incident of Helen's forgetting how to use the control. Until that point, Mike had completely "forgotten" about it. That is to say, he once again repressed the unpleasant awareness that Helen's condition was worsening.

Denial

Denial in the person with Alzheimer's disease, and methods the family should consider in dealing with it, was discussed in the previous chapter. Denial, which is closely related to repression, involves an unwillingness to see, acknowledge, or accept a painful reality. Often, that reality is obvious to others even though it is unrecognized by the individual. Denial can be complete, as exemplified by the wife who simply refuses to acknowledge that her husband, who has had several minor accidents and gotten lost while driving, is no longer able to safely operate a motor vehicle. Denial can also be partial: perhaps the reality is acknowledged, but its significance is denied. For example, the spouse may acknowledge that the individual is forgetful but feels that the items forgotten are not very important, anyway. In this situation, it is not the factual reality (the forgetfulness) that is denied but its emotional implications and importance.

....

Mary Lou and Joseph, both seventy-eight, had been married for more than fifty years. Mary Lou had become increasingly forgetful over the past several years and gradually reached a point where she had great difficulty performing some of her basic activities of daily living. As a result, Joseph helped her to get dressed each morning and undressed at the end of the day. He prepared the meals, cut her food, and often had to help feed her if he served something more complicated than a sandwich or other "finger food." Several times a week, Joseph had to get Mary Lou into the bathtub and wash her. Despite these challenges, Joseph felt that he was managing perfectly well and was not even stressed by the situation. He loved Mary Lou dearly and believed that his commitment to care for her "for better or for worse" was his duty, as she had cared for him and their family for so many years throughout their marriage. His children lived out of state but visited once or twice a month. They were concerned that he was becoming exhausted and would become ill from doing all of these tasks. They noted that he looked drawn and that he had lost a considerable amount of weight over the past year or so. His children, particularly his daughter Carole, urged him to hire someone to help. He considered it but felt that Mary Lou would not like having someone else in the house, so he decided against it. Deep down, he felt it was unnecessary, since he could (and should, he felt) continue the job himself.

....

This example illustrates an important point about defenses in general: it is difficult to determine whether Joseph's attitude regarding the difficulties of caring for Mary Lou represented denial or if it was simply a healthy adaptation to the unpleasant realities of the situation, allowing perhaps for a sense of altruism and a feeling of equanimity. Probably it was a combination of both.

It helps, certainly, to feel that the task is not difficult, but given how exhausted he seemed to the children, and the impact of his providing care on his own health, it would seem that denial was present in addition to altruism. This should serve as a reminder that denial, rather than simply being a troublesome impediment to helping the family member cope effectively, is actually a critical component of human psychic functioning and adaptation that needs to be respected and carefully managed.

It is important to remember that the individual who is using denial is doing so automatically, without any awareness of employing a defense mechanism in order to avoid something unpleasant. Although it may seem otherwise, the person in denial is not doing it "on purpose," in a volitional sense.

Minimization

Minimization consists of acknowledging a reality but convincing oneself that it is less significant, or less severe, than it actually is. In the situation described above, involving Joseph and Mary Lou, Joseph might instead have utilized minimization, feeling that caring for Mary Lou "is a lot of work, but I can manage it without too much trouble," because facing all of the implications of the illness and its impact on himself may be too much for him to endure all at once.

....

Hester and Ralph had been married for more than forty years. They had lived a happy life together. In the past two years, however, Ralph began to show signs of forgetfulness and difficulty with performing tasks. He was ultimately diagnosed with Alzheimer's disease and began treatment with anti-dementia medications. His illness did not improve, but the progression seemed slowed by the medication. Despite his impairments, Ralph continued to drive. He had two small accidents—"fender-benders," he and Hester called them—over the past six months. One of Hester's close friends expressed surprise that Ralph was still driving after these incidents. Hester had concluded that it was still safe for him to drive because the accidents were minor and did not disable the car. It was only after a town policeman stopped him for driving the wrong way around a traffic circle, and revoked his license, that his driving ceased. Hester was no longer able to deal with the situation with minimization, as she had until this point. She was quite relieved that the driving decision was taken out of her hands and that no one had been hurt in the process.

Rationalization

The defense of rationalization uses logical, or pseudological, explanations to justify an action that would otherwise be disturbing or anxiety-provoking. The use of rationalization is akin to the concept of "making excuses," although as with all defenses, the process is unconscious, and the person who rationalizes definitely believes his argument. For example, the family member who uses rationalization as a defense may concede that the person with Alzheimer's does not know the day or month or year but rationalizes this disorientation by claiming that the afflicted individual doesn't *need* to know those things because he is retired. While that may be true, in the strict sense, most individuals who are not impaired cognitively are usually aware of the day of the week, the month, and the year, even if they may not know the precise date of the month. So it may be "rational" not to know these things, but that is beside the point.

....

Bradley had been widowed for more than five years when his growing cognitive impairment led to his moving in to live with his adult daughter, Alberta. This arrangement came about fortuitously, as Bradley's lease was running out and his landlord was raising the rent significantly. Alberta worked as a hairdresser during the day and was able to be home before four in the afternoon most of the time. Bradley, who had become very passive, seemed content to stay home alone by himself, reading, sleeping, watching television, and simply sitting. He did not cook or leave the house, so Alberta felt comfortable with having him there unsupervised during the day.

When she returned home from work, she would typically ask him about his day and if anything special had occurred at home in her absence. Always, the answer was no. On one occasion, Alberta asked if anyone had called on the phone, and Bradley indicated that he thought there might have been a call that afternoon, although he was not able to tell Alberta who had phoned. Alberta asked him to please write down the name and number in the future, and placed a pad and pen next to the telephone. The following day, she again asked if there had been any phone calls, and again Bradley indicated that perhaps someone had called once or twice for Alberta, but he did not know who it was. Clearly, he had forgotten Alberta's request to take a message, or he was not capable of doing so. Rather than again requesting that her father should write a message, or suggesting anything else, she rationalized that if the call was important, the person would try again—with any luck, at a time when she was there to answer the phone herself.

Alberta's rationalization served to avoid any tension with her father over his inability to take messages, which was certainly a good thing, but it did lead to her missing the call from a nearby hair salon to which she had applied for a job some months earlier. At the time she initially applied, they had no openings, but now they were looking for another stylist. They had wanted to offer the job to Alberta, at a somewhat higher salary than she was currently receiving. But they never did call back; she only found out about their offer after she contacted them again, a month or so later, to inquire about openings, and was told how they had tried on several occasions to contact her, unsuccessfully, and had now filled the position.

Avoidance

Avoidance is a common mechanism used by family members, particularly early in the disease process when troubling signs and symptoms begin to appear. In this situation, the person simply avoids having any thoughts about the troublesome issues. If someone else brings it up, the avoidant person may simply change the subject, perhaps without even realizing it.

....

Clyde and Delores had been married for more than forty years. Since Clyde had retired from running the family business about eighteen months earlier, Delores had noted that he was having increasing difficulties with his short-term memory and that he was somewhat more irritable than previously. She initially wrote off these symptoms to the effects of retirement and ignored (that is, denied or minimized) them. However, the situation gradually worsened, and Delores felt an increasing amount of stress overall. At a routine medical appointment, Clyde's physician noted his cognitive difficulties and subsequently performed a cognitive assessment, laboratory studies, and a brain MRI. As a result of his assessment, the physician concluded that Clyde was suffering from Alzheimer's disease and prescribed an anti-dementia medication. He also suggested that Delores obtain *The Thirty-Six Hour Day*, a widely read book for Alzheimer's care partners.

Clyde had a follow-up appointment two months later to review how he was doing with the medication. Delores's son, Fred, accompanied them to the appointment, as he was concerned about his father and did not feel he was able to get a full explanation of what was wrong from his mother. At this appointment, the physician asked Delores if she had obtained *The Thirty-Six Hour Day*, as he had suggested. Delores answered that she had, and that she found it quite interesting and helpful. On the way home from the appointment, Fred asked his mother if he could borrow the book, and Delores indicated that she had "of course" never bought it and that she had no intention of reading such things; she simply did not want to be scolded by the doctor, so she told him her lie about getting it and reading it.

....

Delores's behavior is a clear example of avoidance; she presumably felt that reading a book about Alzheimer's disease would make her more uncomfortable, as she would learn more about the disease and what might be coming in the future. She chose to avoid the discomfort by adopting the stance of not wanting to read about this disease. While she is very aware of making a conscious decision to not buy and read the book, she believes she made this decision because she is too busy to read such material or had no need for it; she is not consciously aware of her desire to avoid it because its content would make her too uncomfortable.

Displacement

The defense of displacement involves focusing on one idea in order to avoid coming to grips with another. For example, it may be easier for a spouse to focus anxiously on trying to keep the house orderly rather than to feel overwhelmed by the disorder created by the disease.

....

Mel and Gloria were in their early seventies. A second marriage for both, they had been together for more than thirty years and had a very close relationship. Gloria noticed that Mel was beginning to forget events from the recent past and was becoming quite repetitive. She tried to ignore this initially, but the symptoms appeared to worsen. Finally, one of her stepsons visited and seemed alarmed at the changes he noted in his father. He asked Gloria to have Mel evaluated. She arranged for Mel to be seen by a highly regarded neurologist for assessment of his cognitive impairment. At the end of the appointment, the doctor rather coldly told Mel and Gloria that Mel was suffering from Alzheimer's disease and that it would continually worsen over the next several years, at which point Mel would likely need a nursing home. The doctor indicated that that he would send a report to Mel's primary doctor with this information. With that, he abruptly left the room, ending the appointment. Both Mel and Gloria were understandably angered by the way this was handled, and talked on the way home about the doctor's abrupt, unfeeling style, rather than the diagnosis he had given.

But Mel and Gloria both used the defense of displacement, focusing on the doctor's cold manner in order to keep from having to squarely face the bad news he had delivered.

Emotions as Defenses

Some emotions are less painful for the family member to face than others, and thus emotions can be used defensively as well. For example, it may be easier for a family member to feel angry toward the afflicted loved one because of his apathy or disengagement, rather than recognizing that the disease has robbed him of being able to show any initiative. The use of emotions in this defensive manner are discussed in more detail in the following chapter.

Intellectualization

Intellectualization helps to reduce anxiety by causing the individual to avoid dwelling on the stressful, anxiety-provoking aspect of something unpleasant and instead to focus only on the more factual, dispassionate aspects of it.

....

Eleanor had been increasingly forgetful for about one year. Her husband, Bob, was very concerned with how she seemed more vague and confused when she slept poorly. Bob made a chart of hours slept plotted against numbers of cognitive errors made per day, and brought this to Eleanor's clinic appointment. He also pored over the medical literature on sleep and cognition in order to intellectually "prove" that the problem was insomnia, not Alzheimer's disease. Although sleep was indeed a concern for Eleanor, she did, in fact have Alzheimer's disease of mild to moderate severity.

....

Intellectualization, like other defenses, can be a helpful coping strategy, as well, when used appropriately. For example, a person who has just been diagnosed with a very serious illness might focus on learning everything about the disease, rather than only the emotional implications of it. There can be value in this approach, not just to ease the emotional impact of facing such a serious illness, but also because having more knowledge about a disease is certainly helpful in partnering with the physician who will treat it. This applies to Alzheimer's disease, as well, although it is usually the family member and not the person with the disease whose intellectualization can be put to a valuable use. Learning as much as possible about the illness certainly helps family members cope more effectively with having a loved one with the disease. Becoming very knowledgeable about the disease is extremely important for family members. But it is a matter of *how* this intellectual information is used: on the one hand, it can be used to help family members get closer to the subjective experience of the person with the disease as well as their own reactions to it. On the other hand, intellectual information can be used to create an emotional distance or barrier between the family and the person with the disease, by avoiding the emotional implications of the situation. Health-care professionals are particularly vulnerable to defensive, excessive use of intellectualization when dealing with medical problems in themselves or a loved one.

Compartmentalization

Compartmentalization is a defense that can be a valuable coping strategy—for example, the husband who simply decides not to think about his wife's illness while busy at work, putting his worries about the situation in a mental "compartment" that is not opened while he is at work. Although this can certainly be useful, excessive compartmentalizing can easily lead to complete avoidance of the problem emotionally. Once again, the important issue is *how* the defense mechanism is used, more than simply the fact that a defense mechanism is at work.

The Positive Value of Defensive Functioning

It is important to emphasize once again that the use of a particular defense mechanism is not automatically pathological, something to be confronted and broken down as soon as it is identified. In fact, defenses play a very necessary role in daily life. They can be thought of as psychological "shock absorbers" which keep the daily ride a bit smoother, as the painful emotional bumps and potholes that would otherwise be so jarring are encountered. The use of defense mechanisms can help the family face more gradually, over time, the extremely painful emotions that having a loved one with Alzheimer's brings. Everyone uses defenses in this way, not just Alzheimer's families.

....

Bill did not have Alzheimer's disease or any other cognitive disorder. He was recently told by his physician that a growth on his skin is likely cancerous, although the definitive diagnosis would come from the biopsy report in a few days. While waiting for the biopsy results, Bill used a variety of defenses in an understandable attempt to cope with the frightening implications of this news. For example, he initially felt that because the physician did not say that the growth was definitely cancer, it probably was not. This is a form of denial. Later, Bill came to feel that, because he has had no pain, the growth probably was not serious, or could be easily cured. This is an example of rationalization at work. Bill also went on the Internet and read as much as he could about the type of skin lesion he had. This was an intellectualization at work, since learning about the disease and its treatments helped to reduce Bill's anxiety.

....

One can certainly appreciate that Bill utilized these defenses to protect himself from having to face, all at once, the likelihood of having cancer. The judicious use of certain defenses, particularly denial and rationalization, can help an individual maintain a critical sense of hope and optimism in the face of bad news.

Pathological Use of Defenses

Although defenses can be helpful, their excessive, rigid, or otherwise inappropriate use can be problematic. A defense should be viewed as undesirable or pathological when its use leads to some type of disadvantage or harm to the individual. Consider, once again, Bill and his skin lesion. If, after learning that the biopsy confirmed that his lesion was cancerous, Bill had decided not to proceed with any treatment, because he believed the biopsy report to be wrong, this would represent potentially dangerous defensive thinking that we would label as pathological denial. If, on the other hand, after receiving the biopsy results, Bill told himself that he would call the physician the next day to schedule an appointment to discuss treatment, but somehow did not remember to make the call for several weeks, this might be considered an example of a pathologic degree of repression. Fortunately, Bill did neither of these things; he called his physician to schedule an appointment for treatment the same day he received the biopsy result that the lesion was, unfortunately, cancerous. Once confronted with the unambiguous biopsy report, he was able to put aside his denial, rationalization, and intellectualization, and address the problem in the most appropriate fashion.

....

Alice has Alzheimer's disease, recently diagnosed. Harley, her husband, noted that Alice had been driving much too close to the center line, often changed lanes without signaling, and had dented the car's bumper by hitting a parking meter. Rather than recognize these behaviors as an indication that Alice's driving should at least be evaluated, if not stopped, Harley used the defense of rationalization to avoid facing the situation. He explained to himself that her poor driving was a result of their having purchased a new car less than a year earlier, and that it is wider than their previous one. Harley hoped her driving would improve, and simply asked Alice to "be more careful." A week later, Alice made a right turn from the left-hand lane and did not signal. Her car was hit on the passenger side by a vehicle traveling in the right lane. Thankfully, no one was seriously injured, but both vehicles suffered significant damage. At that point, Harley asked that Alice give up driving for good, and although she did not agree that was necessary (when reminded of her accident, she insisted that it was the other driver's fault), she reluctantly acquiesced.

....

It should be clear from this example that while defenses are often employed out of an understandable desire not to face the unpleasant realities of a situation, this can lead to serious negative consequences if the defenses don't readily yield to the demands of reality. It is to be hoped that harm does not have to come to the person with Alzheimer's, or to others, for the family member to recognize a defense mechanism being used to dangerous excess. But there are times when a defense mechanism can assume a too-powerful, automatic, or rigid role in the coping style of the family member, so that the realities of the situation are never acknowledged or accepted. Even (or perhaps especially) when defenses are used with great rigidity, they may not completely prevent anxiety or other difficult feelings from reaching awareness. Therefore, the family member who is overly defensive may appear anxious or depressed, although he may not acknowledge these feelings. The family member who is pathologically defensive will not make optimal decisions regarding the person with Alzheimer's disease. This may have been the case for Harley concerning Alice and her driving.

The Repeated Appearance of Defenses

Defenses do not arise in a neat, orderly fashion, to be dealt with and put to rest forever, one at a time. Defenses can and usually will arise repeatedly, depending on the current circumstances. For example, recognizing that one has been in denial about the memory difficulties of a loved one doesn't mean that denial will never occur again.

....

Ruth was initially in denial that her mother, Claudia, was impaired in any way, despite Claudia's obvious short-term memory and functional difficulties. She simply attributed the memory difficulty to aging and poor hearing. Eventually, it became apparent that Claudia was neglecting to pay her monthly bills, and the telephone was disconnected for a brief period of time until Ruth intervened with the phone company and took care of the overdue bill. In addition, Claudia frequently repeated questions whenever Ruth would visit. Ruth finally recognized that something was, indeed, wrong; the severity of Claudia's symptoms overpowered Ruth's denial. Ruth was able to acknowledge to herself that Claudia had a cognitive problem and took her to the doctor, who diagnosed her dementia. But as the disease gradually worsened, Ruth again used denial in order not to face new elements of the situation that were developing. For some time Ruth denied that Claudia had progressed to such a degree that she should no longer be left alone, despite the continuing advance of symptoms. However, when Ruth described Claudia's condition at the first support group she attended, other support group members helped her realize that she was in denial regarding the seriousness of the situation and emphasized that she needed to act in order to ensure Claudia's safety. Having this pointed out to her in a nonjudgmental fashion by others who were in a very similar situation allowed Ruth to understand and accept the fact that she was not wishing to see the severity of Claudia's illness.

As a result of this awareness, she was able to change her attitude. Ruth promptly arranged for someone to come to the house daily, which her mother actually accepted quite readily.

....

Ruth and Claudia's situation makes clear that as each new symptom or dysfunction develops, there can be a recurrence of denial or other defenses. However, recognizing and working through a particular defense mechanism when it first appears can sometimes make it easier to recognize and manage it when it appears again, particularly if the family member is open-minded about the process. Other family members, or friends familiar with the situation, may be quite helpful as well. It is common that others will become aware of the defensive nature of a particular behavior or attitude before the individual, herself, will. This is, of course, similar to the situation with the denial in the person with Alzheimer's disease: usually, family members will be more aware of the person's illness than he is.

The example of Ruth and Claudia also makes clear the enormous value of attending a support group. This is discussed in more detail in chapter 7.

The Value of Lessening Defenses in Family Members

Because the family member uses defenses to avoid, delay, or lessen the emotional impact of the disease, it is likely that as his defenses begin to lessen, he will become increasingly aware of a variety of difficult emotions he has concerning the person with the illness. Going through the painful process of lessening defenses is not only necessary and inevitable but, ultimately, valuable for both the family member and the person with Alzheimer's. Becoming less defensive helps the family member face more directly the realities of the illness and therefore to make more appropriate decisions regarding care.

Mary's daughter, Julia, was in denial about Mary's illness and rationalized that Mary's moderately advanced Alzheimer's was only a mild affliction. She felt it was still safe for Mary to live alone, even though there had been clear indications that this was no longer a wise option. Mary was losing weight, eating little, and there was often spoiled food in the refrigerator that Julia had brought over weeks earlier. Mary was quite erratic about taking her pills, skipping them for days at a time, but also, on more than one occasion, taking at least two days' pills on a single day. In addition, the house was in considerable disarray. On one of Julia's visits, she noted that the cat's food dish was filled with kitty litter rather than cat food. Julia's defensive self-distortions about the safety of the situation were certainly understandable, given her deep love for Mary and her lifelong admiration for Mary's considerable intelligence and independence. But Julia's denial began to break down when Mary had to be hospitalized with a severe gastrointestinal illness brought about either by improper use of medication or eating spoiled food, or both. This event led Julia to realize that her mother could no longer live alone, and after her hospitalization and a brief period at a rehabilitation center, Julia brought Mary to live with her and began the process of selling Mary's house.

In every Alzheimer's family, there are examples of the family learning "the hard way" that the disease is worse than suspected, or worse than they allowed themselves to recognize. A family member's defenses can sometimes be broken through abruptly as a result of an untoward event, as was the case for Mary and Julia. But it should be clear that there is less likelihood of harm and less turmoil for both the person with the disease and the family if defenses are reduced and the situation is seen more clearly before a serious adverse event occurs, rather than only afterward. Of course, this is not to say that all undesirable occurrences are the result of the family's defensiveness—far from it. The nature of Alzheimer's disease is such that unexpected and unwelcome incidents will inevitably arise in every Alzheimer's family. But a family member who is able to see the situation accurately and objectively, rather than through the distorting lens of psychological defenses, will be best equipped to lessen the risk of adverse events and to appropriately manage those that do occur.

How Family Defenses Become Reduced

How do the family member's defenses get broken down? There are several ways this happens. First, as the disease inexorably progresses, the realities of the illness will strike at family members repeatedly, slowly lessening defenses as if by erosion. While this will eventually prove effective, it can take a great deal of time and can be painful—and potentially dangerous—for both the family and the person with Alzheimer's. This was the case for Harley and Alice concerning her driving; it took a major accident for Harley's denial to be broken down sufficiently for him to realize the necessity that Alice cease driving.

Learning about the illness, along with the emotional issues that families typically face, is another tool that helps break down defenses. This can occur by reading books, attending lectures, reviewing the many valuable sites about Alzheimer's disease on the Internet, and so forth. Replacing the defenses of repression, denial, rationalization, and minimization with knowledge (and sometimes even a degree of intellectualization) can move the family member closer to facing the situation realistically. While intellectual insight alone may not be sufficient to break down firmly held defenses, it can help the family member recognize her own responses to the disease, if she is open to such self-knowledge.

It may also be helpful for the individual to work through these issues with a therapist who is skilled in treating family members of persons with Alzheimer's disease. This would be especially true for a family member who has difficulty seeing her own role in the

Alzheimer's process or for one who is in a great deal of distress over the situation. Many family members are quite reluctant to pursue therapy or counseling. This seems to be particularly true for older persons. It also seems that those family members who could most benefit from therapy are often the most resistant to it. At any rate, many family members seem to prefer to deal with these issues on their own or with the help of other family members, friends, clergy, the primary doctor, or others. This can be quite useful, particularly if the helper has some previous experience in dealing with Alzheimer's disease.

Finally, attending an Alzheimer's support group can be one of the most valuable tools for dealing with the family member's defenses. This was certainly true for Ruth, who had difficulty seeing that her mother, Claudia, was no longer safe at home alone until this was nonjudgmentally pointed out to her in her first support group meeting. Support groups help with the many psychological and emotional challenges family members face, as well the practical issues that arise when one has a loved one with Alzheimer's disease. Enormous benefits can come from expressing one's feelings to others who are coping with very similar issues and who don't make value judgments about the feelings expressed. Support group members can offer meaningful feedback and positive suggestions that are often more readily accepted than the advice of professionals. All Alzheimer's family members should attend a support group, even (perhaps especially) those who feel they don't "need" it. Support groups are discussed in greater detail in chapter 7.

The Transition to Higher-Level Defenses

Once the family member has largely set aside her defenses and resolved some of the other emotional challenges that can occur, and after confronting and dealing with the core emotional issue of grief that then comes to the surface, the processes of adaptation, acceptance, and moving forward can begin. Of course, the emotions generated by living with someone with this disease are no less distressing at this point than they were earlier, but a series of "higher-level" defenses can now be employed by the family member to help cope with these issues in more positive ways. This is discussed at more length in the final chapter of this book.

Chapter Three

Common Emotions Experienced by the Family Care Partner

This chapter focuses on several common emotional reactions that family members may feel when coping with a loved one who has Alzheimer's: anxiety, guilt, anger, and shame. In chapter 5, grief, the emotion that is at the center of the family member's journey, will be examined in depth.

Not every family member experiences anxiety, guilt, anger, or shame to the same degree, of course; these feelings may be experienced at different times and with different intensities by different family care partners, according to the particulars of the situation and the personality of the family member. And there can be other emotions that family members will have in the course of caring for a loved one with Alzheimer's disease, as well. But these four, along with grief, are the most common, and most difficult, emotions that family members experience.

What about Depression?

Depression, in the common, nonclinical use of the term, is nearly universal in family members caring for someone with Alzheimer's. It is part of the grief response that lies at the center of the family care partner's journey. Depression, in the clinical sense of the word, can be seen as a complication of the stress of providing care, particularly for the vulnerable family member. It has a number of features that differentiate it from "simple" sadness. Despair, which consists of depression with significant hopelessness, may be common in family members who are unable to reach the stage of acceptance. These considerations are discussed in more detail in chapters 7 and 8.

Anxiety, guilt, anger, and shame can be very powerful, very pervasive, and very painful. But, despite their importance, these emotions lie *outside* the central emotional experience of the Alzheimer's family member, which consists of grief over the gradual loss of the loved one. As important or pervasive as these feelings may be, they nevertheless can stand in the way of the family member's full experience of grief. In that sense they resemble defense mechanisms, and at times they do function defensively, as was mentioned in the previous chapter. This is not to say that these emotions are artificial or intentionally concocted in any way. They are very real emotions, indeed, and are based on the interplay of the particular features of the person with Alzheimer's, the history of the particular family relationships involved, and the family member's underlying personality. But in order to fully face and eventually come to terms with the grief that loved ones feel, it is necessary to understand these difficult emotions, work through them, and then delve into the emotional core of grief.

As noted above, not every family member experiences each of these emotions with the same intensity. But the more a family member is preoccupied with these feelings, the more this will interfere with facing and coming to terms with the core issue of grief.

Anxiety

It was mentioned in chapter 2 that one of the chief motivations for defensive behavior is to lessen or avoid anxiety. So it is not surprising that, as the family member's defenses are lessened, anxiety increases (Cooper et al. 2006). The primary source of this anxiety is that the immediate and long-term future is unknown. All that is known with certainty is that the disease will continue, and continue to worsen, with or without treatment, until death.

But many critical questions that family members ask themselves cannot be answered with any degree of certainty or accuracy.

- What symptoms will develop in the near future?
- How long will she be able to remain living at home?
- Will I be able to handle the stresses that arise?
- Can I manage all of the tasks that he was doing—for example, handling the finances, fixing things that break around the house, doing the shopping and cooking?
- Can we continue to travel?
- Will she continue to know who I am?
- Will he become violent toward me?
- How do I handle the various behaviors that arise?
- Can she be left alone even for a short while or must someone always be present?
- Will I know if and when it is time to put him in a nursing home?
- If a nursing home becomes necessary, can we afford it?
- Will there be anything left for me to live on, or to leave to the children?

In more conflicted relationships, other critical questions may arise—for example:

- Do I want to be a care partner, giving up my independence and freedom in order to care for this person for the indefinite future?
- Would he (or she) take care of me if the roles were reversed?
- What if I find I don't want to do it any longer—can I quit?

When the primary family member is an adult child, still other questions are likely to occur—namely:

- How do I take adequate care of my parent and still meet my obligations to my spouse and my own children?
- Should I move my parent into our house?

- How will this affect my relationship with my spouse?
- How will this affect my relationship with my children?
- Do I need to give up my job in order to adequately care for my parent?

This is just a small sampling of the kinds of questions that family members must face when a loved one is diagnosed with Alzheimer's. Many of these questions will arise repeatedly throughout the illness. The element of uncertainty about exactly how, and how rapidly, the illness will progress deprives the care partner of a critical tool for coping with an anxiety-provoking situation—planning. Even though some advance planning can (and should) be undertaken, because it is known that the disease will be incurable and progressive, there remains a great amount of uncertainty about the particular course that anyone's illness will take.

How does this anxiety manifest itself? Because of the reciprocal relationship between anxiety and defensiveness, it is possible that the family member will (unconsciously, of course) attempt to control his anxiety with a renewed reliance on defenses. The family member who feels overwhelmed by the growing dependence of the person with the disease may, for example, begin to feel that the person with Alzheimer's really *can* do more for herself, but simply doesn't *want* to—a good example of rationalization at work. This will only lead to frustration and anger at the victim, but in the family member's personal emotional equation, those feelings may be more tolerable than the anxiety that her dependence otherwise engenders. When the defenses give way to the unpleasant current reality, a greater sense of apprehension may take over, along with sleep problems, difficulty concentrating, somatic concerns, panic attacks, general fears, overuse of alcohol or other mood-altering substances, and so forth. Other behaviors may appear in the family member—for example, a tendency to hover overprotectively around the person with the disease and to actually prevent her from having even that degree of autonomy that she could manage, for fear of an untoward event occurring.

....

Ann and Tom were married for more than fifty years, prior to Ann's death from a heart attack. Although family members were aware that Tom had shown some degree of forgetfulness, Ann (who had no cognitive impairment) was able to manage his needs very well and thus to mask the difficulties he was having. Only when she died, did it become apparent how much Tom had relied on her for cognitive support.

Tom and Ann had three children, Ben, Leon, and Ginger. Ginger lived the closest and was not married, and so it fell to her to look after her father. Ginger had long believed that her father favored her siblings, Ben and Leon, over her, because they were males, and married, and she was not. After Ann's death, more tension developed between them. Ginger noted that her father was not able to discern the day of the week or keep track of any appointments. He was able to do some basic meal preparation, but while she was alive, Ann had done the grocery shopping and all of the cooking. Tom was able to dress himself, but Ginger noticed that he now wore the same outfits for many days in a row, and they were often wrinkled or food-stained. Initially, Ginger attributed her father's difficulties to his understandable grief over Ann's death, and she was glad to assist him, even moving into her father's home temporarily, after Ann's death.

However, after a few months, Tom's cognitive difficulties were certainly no better, and in fact seemed worse, although it may simply be that Ginger's closer presence in his life enabled her to see more of the difficulties that had been present for some time. Ginger came to feel that her father had become too dependent on Ann for his daily tasks and that he was now trying to transfer that "unhealthy dependency," as she called it, onto her. Ginger felt that Tom was capable of doing more independently but did not *want* to do so, preferring to have Ginger take care of him instead. As a result, Ginger became impatient with her father and talked about moving back to her own apartment. Tom suggested that she continue to live there with him, to save the cost of her apartment rental—and because he probably recognized his need to have her there, although he did not want to admit this either to Ginger or to himself. Nevertheless, Ginger moved back to her own place, believing that this would be best for them both. But Ginger felt uneasy about this decision, wondering if she had done the right thing, and often lay awake at night worrying about her father, feeling angry with him for his dependency, and missing her mother.

Within a few weeks, it became clear that Ginger's hope that Tom would be more capable of independent functioning if he were "forced" to be on his own was not going to be realized. Tom became more disheveled, ate poorly, and probably did not bathe once during the time Ginger was away. He missed an appointment with his primary care physician and his weekly card game with his friends at the Legion Hall. When Ginger visited, bringing food and some cooked meals to Tom, she also determined that Tom had missed many days' worth of medications. Ginger noted all of this with alarm and with a great deal of anxiety. She called Ben and Leon, who both lived out of town with their own families, to discuss how to handle the situation. Ben and Leon recognized that Tom should not live alone, and encouraged Ginger to move in with him permanently, in order to care for him. Ginger felt overwhelmed at the responsibility they were suggesting she assume, but her immediate response was to feel anger at her siblings for "dumping" this situation on her and envious that they had their own lives and families and were thus "excused," at least in their own minds, from the task of parental care. Ginger loved her own apartment and greatly valued her job in a bank office, which so far had been generous and understanding of her need for time off to care for her father. In addition, it was Ginger's hope that as she pursued her single lifestyle, she would eventually meet someone to marry. She was now in her mid-thirties, and she felt that if she had to give up her apartment to move back home with her father, she would probably lose, forever, the chance to find a partner. She saw herself becoming an angry and sad old maid who lived at home with her father.

Despite these difficult feelings, Ginger did move back in with her father, telling Tom and herself that this was just temporary, while Tom "got back on his feet," but she was increasingly doubtful that would ever happen. She went to her job during the day but rushed home right after work to cook dinner and take care of Tom. She felt a great deal of anxiety, thinking about the situation, and at times this translated again into resentment and denial, thinking again that her father could be doing more for himself if he hadn't become so dependent, initially, on his wife. She continued to feel anger toward her siblings. She wondered if she should put her father in a care facility but rejected that idea because she believed that her father was not sufficiently impaired for that, and also because her father had more than once said "at least I still have our home"; now that Ann was no longer living, he felt her presence in the house they had shared for so many years, and he was comforted by that. Ginger lay awake at night mulling the situation over, wondering how long it would go on, and ultimately decided to go to her doctor for medication to help her sleep, as her fatigue and anxiety were beginning to interfere with her performance at work. Her doctor recommended she return to a therapist she had seen after a relationship ended several years ago, in order to help her sort out the new issues and responsibilities in her life and to cope with the considerable anxiety and uncertainty she was experiencing.

....

What should the anxious family member do about these difficult feelings? The first step, as always, is to recognize their presence, and to understand how denial and other defenses may have been working to lessen their impact. It is then important for the family member to try to understand—by herself, with the help of a trusted confidante, or a therapist—exactly what it is about the situation that is causing the greatest degree of anxiety. Many family members would say that the whole situation is causing their anxiety, and while there is truth in that, of course, it is helpful to try to understand the specific origins of the anxiety in more detail. In Ginger's case, her anxiety had to do with being faced with her father's growing cognitive impairment and resultant dependency, and her feeling that it was going to be she, largely by herself, that would need to deal with it. That thought seemed open-ended and overwhelming to her, as reflected in her middle-of-the-night ruminations that she would end up living with her father forever. Beyond that, her anxiety also signaled her increasing fears that she would never meet someone to marry. As she worked on this in her therapy, she realized that living with her father did not preclude her forming a relationship, and that if she wanted to have some evenings free for dating or other activities, she could arrange for someone to come to stay with him for those hours. She also realized in therapy that, behind all of these concerns was her deep sadness at the thought of gradually losing her father to this illness, particularly so soon after the death of her mother.

Another important way to decrease the anxiety of having a loved one with Alzheimer's is to learn as much as possible about the disease, through reading, lectures, the Internet, and, especially, through attending a support group. While this won't give the family member the ability to know exactly how the situation will unfold, it will certainly help lessen the feelings of being anxious and overwhelmed by the uncertainties of the disease. The value of attending a support group is discussed further in chapter 7.

Guilt

It is very common for family members to struggle with feelings of guilt regarding their loved one's illness (Martin et al. 2006). The degree to which this is experienced may have at least as much to do with the family member's underlying personality as it does with the realities of the disease itself. For example, a spouse who has been prone to feeling guilty throughout life in a wide variety of situations will, not surprisingly, tend to be burdened with a great deal of guilt in regard to his spouse's illness and how well he is providing care.

Guilt is certainly an emotion that nearly everyone has experienced, to a greater or lesser degree. It is normal to feel some amount of guilt when one has knowingly violated a law or a social custom, or done something that causes harm or offense to another person. To *not* experience feelings of guilt occasionally—to have no "conscience"—is a serious character flaw that is associated with sociopathic personalities, hardened criminals, and the like. On the other hand, the opposite situation—being burdened with feelings of guilt when one has committed no offense—is unfortunately very common. Wrestling with unnecessary guilt causes untold amounts of personal suffering. Mental health professionals note that pervasive but inappropriate feelings of guilt are among the most common reasons for which individuals seek counseling or psychotherapy.

How, and why, do family members of people with Alzheimer's disease experience feelings of guilt about the illness, and how does it affect them and the person with the disease? Certainly, most family members know that they have done nothing to cause the disease. Nevertheless, some guilt-prone family members—particularly spouses—may harbor these beliefs, especially if there has been some ambivalence or other difficulties throughout the relationship. Others may have long-standing, but unresolved, feelings of culpability about aspects of their conduct in the marriage, and when Alzheimer's appears, it becomes the displaced focus of that guilt.

....

Victoria and Harold had been married for forty-five years. On the surface, all seemed well, but for years Harold had been frustrated by what he felt was Victoria's emotional reserve and lack of sexual interest and responsiveness. More than twenty-five years earlier, Harold developed an attraction to Rachel, a female coworker, and after several months of casual office flirtation, they went out for drinks after work one night and ended up having a sexual encounter. Their sexual liaison was repeated on two more occasions over the next six months. At that point, Rachel took a position across the country, and they never saw each other again. Harold felt saddened yet also relieved by her moving away and wrestled for years with uncomfortable feelings about his extramarital behavior. He never told Victoria about the affair with Rachel. He obviously felt guilty, but he justified his actions by telling himself that no one was hurt and that it was his way of coping with Victoria's lack of sexual appetite. He loved her very much, despite this, and never repeated the behavior with anyone else. Eventually he put the affair aside, mentally, and stopped thinking about it.

Years later, when Victoria developed Alzheimer's, Harold understandably felt great anguish. He became extraordinarily attentive to her needs and seemed to relish all of the chores he took over from her and the many tasks involved in her care. After eight years of active illness, Victoria had reached the later stages of disease. At that point, their children began to express concern for Harold's own failing health. They repeatedly urged him to place her in a nursing home, for his own well-being, but he strongly resisted the idea. Even though she progressed to a point of not knowing where she was and not usually recognizing Harold, he felt that placement was not necessary, and he simply would not consider it.

Unfortunately, several months into his ninth year of caring for Victoria, Harold fell down a flight of stairs at home while heading to the kitchen to get lunch for her, and he fractured his left hip and forearm. His hospitalization and subsequent rehabilitation stay forced Harold to reluctantly accept his family's and the doctors' recommendation that Victoria be placed in long-term care, as it was unclear when, if ever, he would be well enough to resume caring for her at home. Nevertheless, Harold felt enormous guilt about the placement. He had promised Victoria years earlier that he would never put her in a facility, and now he had broken that promise.

It was only later, some time after Victoria died in the nursing home that Harold, still feeling guilty, recognized that he could not have possibly continued to care for her at home after his accident. For the first time, he talked to his physician about his affair with Rachel so many years earlier, and he recognized that his guilt over that episode came back to the surface with Victoria's diagnosis. He felt proud of the job he did as care partner for so long but realized that some of his zeal for providing care came from a need or desire to "atone" for his actions of the past. On some level, he felt that his transgression and perhaps his conflicted feelings during that period in their marriage had somehow contributed to Victoria's developing Alzheimer's. Even as he said this, he recognized the absurdity of it, but still had difficulty shaking the feeling.

....

The story of Harold and Victoria brings up several important points. One is the long-lasting and often partially hidden nature of guilt. Harold's guilt was caused, or intensified, by his relationship with Rachel more than a quarter of a century earlier. Guilt is sometimes most readily discovered not by the subjective emotions (which may be hidden even from the guilt-ridden one) but by the *behaviors* that it seems to drive, in order to avoid or lessen the guilt feelings. While Harold's attentiveness toward Victoria's illness was certainly exemplary, it is interesting to note that Harold himself felt that at least some of the motivation for this behavior was related to his long-standing feelings of guilt.

Many family care partners continue to make daily visits to the nursing home after the person with Alzheimer's has long ceased to recognize the immediate family. While there may be a variety of motivations that determine this behavior, a common one is to avoid feeling guilty for "abandoning" the loved one in the facility. The well spouse feels that because she *can* visit, she *must* visit—there is no excuse to do otherwise. These family members may not initially recognize that their daily visit is being driven by wanting to avoid feelings of guilt, but they will often acknowledge (reluctantly) that when bad weather or a cold forces them to avoid the nursing home for a day or two, they are glad to have a "legitimate" reason not to visit and are able to enjoy a day to themselves.

Another point to be emphasized from the story of Harold and Victoria is the risk of promising to never place a loved one in a nursing home. While the sentiment is certainly laudable, it is obviously not possible to foresee the need for nursing home care before the disease even begins, or when it is in its earliest stages, which is often when these promises are made. However, if and when the time comes that placement must be considered, that promise can lead to behaviors that are driven as much, or more, by wanting to avoid guilt (not wanting to break the promise) as by more realistic considerations. It is not clear how much this promise caused Harold to reject his children's pleas to place Victoria, and how much had to do with his continuing need to expiate his guilt from his affair years earlier, or other factors.

While guilt rarely causes a family member to act in ways that are overtly harmful to the loved one with Alzheimer's, it can cause missed opportunities for positive experiences.

....

Ervin and Linda had been married for more than fifty years, and Ervin had suffered from Alzheimer's disease for about two years. Linda cared for him at home but had been feeling stressed by having less and less time to herself as Ervin's needs increased. Through an ad in the local paper, she became aware of an adult day program in the next town. She considered it for Ervin, but put it aside for several months, feeling that Ervin probably would not want to go and that it was selfish of her to want to take him just so she could have some time to herself, anyway. Nevertheless, with the urging of Ervin's physician, Linda decided to try out the program, arranging for him to stay for just the morning on his first day. She left him there with some trepidation and no small amount of guilt. She drove around aimlessly for some time, thinking about the situation, then finally went home and essentially did nothing but watch the clock until it was time to pick him up again at the center. When she returned to get him, Ervin was mildly agitated and repeatedly asked Linda where she had gone. She felt terribly guilty for putting him through this, and when she asked if he wanted to go again the following week, he said that he did not. Although the program director indicated that he seemed to do well and had only become anxious near the end of the morning, she never again brought him to the program.

....

It is certainly common that someone with Alzheimer's will react negatively to the first visit at a day program, but with some gentle but persistent urging he can often be persuaded to try it again. With repeated visits, people like Ervin may find that they actually enjoy the program, which would be a valuable opportunity for socialization and functioning outside the home. Linda seemed to give up on the day program too soon, not wanting to feel guilty for making Ervin do something he initially didn't seem to want to do; thus she may have deprived him of a positive activity in his life. In addition, she deprived herself of a good opportunity for some time to herself.

Other family members avoid pursuing friendships or other activities outside the home. They may rationalize this behavior by stating that it simply is too hard to make the necessary arrangements for care. While it can be difficult to do this, it is rarely impossible if there are funds available to hire someone to be with the person or if there are other family or friends available to help.

Many will resist the idea of asking an adult child to spend time with the parent, feeling that the children "have their own lives" and should not be burdened with this task. However, except in truly dysfunctional families, adult children are usually quite willing to help if they are able, even if they often find it very easy to simply "let Mom do it." On closer examination, many of these family care partners, particularly spouses, will acknowledge that they would feel too guilty if they were to pursue a pleasurable activity outside the home. They feel that if their spouse is unable to enjoy this type of activity, they should not, either.

....

Martha cared for her husband, Louis, at home. Louis was diagnosed with Alzheimer's disease three years ago. Martha was six years younger than Louis and in excellent health. Prior to Louis's illness she regularly attended a monthly book group with about ten of her friends. However, as her husband's disease progressed and his needs for care and monitoring increased, Martha stopped going to the book group meetings. Initially she blamed this on not having time to read the assigned books, although the group was quite casual about that expectation, and there were always several members at each meeting who had not finished (or sometimes even started) the book. She then felt that it was simply too complicated to arrange for someone to stay with Louis. Her daughter-in-law, who lived locally, offered to come over and be with Louis so she could go, but Martha felt reluctant to "burden" her in this way.

Martha was able to get herself to go to the book group only after a discussion about this in her Alzheimer's support group helped her to understand the reason for her reluctance: she felt too guilty to do something enjoyable while her beloved husband was unable to share in this pleasure. Louis had previously been an avid reader, and in fact, years earlier, had been the one to encourage her to join the book group in the first place. Although he never attended the meetings, he used to read the books that the group assigned, and he and Martha would discuss these at home prior to the book group's meetings. He often had insights about the book that had eluded her. But as his disease progressed, he became less and less able to comprehend what he read and finally gave up reading completely. Only when Martha was able to recognize how needlessly remorseful she felt and realized that Louis undoubtedly would want her to continue to go and enjoy this activity, was she able to put aside her guilt and resume attending the meetings. But she would always leave right at the end of the session and rush home, not milling around as some of the others did to socialize for another fifteen to twenty minutes.

....

Family members who feel a strong sense of guilt are often outstanding care partners; but their suffering in the process certainly does not help the person with the disease, or anyone else, including themselves. These devoted family members may need to be reminded that the most important gift they can give their loved one is to do whatever is necessary to maximize the likelihood that they will be available to them for the duration of their illness. The best way to ensure this is for the family member to take proper care of herself. This includes looking after her physical health and emotional well-being. Care partners who do not do this may end up too ill or too emotionally overwhelmed to continue. Attending to one's own emotional well-being requires that the family member have adequate periods of respite, regular opportunities to see friends, to pursue other interests, and simply to engage in activities that do not involve providing care. There are some family members—most commonly but not exclusively older wives—for whom the frequently given advice of "take care of yourself" is generally unhelpful, because these individuals have always felt that focusing on one's own needs is inappropriate, self-indulgent, and to be eschewed. For these guilt-driven and duty-driven family members, it is necessary to point out that they must attend, however reluctantly, to their own needs so that they will be fit and available to carry out their care-providing "duties" for as long as possible.

Decreasing the sense of guilt that drives so many family members can be a significant challenge. It is important for family members to realize that this type of guilt, when no offense has been committed, is a completely unnecessary and a quietly destructive emotion. Sometimes it can be viewed as a form of "survivor guilt"—the individual is spared while others, sometimes but not always family members, become victims. Those who survived a house fire or car accident, an infectious outbreak such as polio in the 1950s, or the horrors of the Holocaust are often severely emotionally crippled by survivor guilt, and no amount of appeal to rational thinking can ease their lifelong burden of culpability over having lived through what others have not. While the situation with Alzheimer's may not be the same as these examples, the emotional state in which the "surviving" family member finds himself can be quite similar and just as intractable.

Anger

Nearly every involved family member will experience anger toward the person with Alzheimer's occasionally (Tabak et al. 1997). Whether this is in reaction to the repetitive questions that are so much a part of the illness, or in response to other particular behaviors, or simply in response to frustration with the overall situation, feelings of anger, and their occasional overt expression, are ubiquitous. After feeling and especially after expressing anger, many family members will experience strong pangs of regret. While feeling excessive remorse over the occasional sharp retort to a repetitive question has more to do with guilt than with anger, most family members feel bad about it, recognize that they should have kept their moment of temper to themselves, tell themselves to avoid doing it in the future, but do not dwell on it.

It is expected that most family members will, at least at some point in their journey with Alzheimer's, feel furious that this disease has occurred in their lives. This may be especially true for spouses, who may understandably feel that they have been robbed of the peaceful, satisfying later years of their life, which they have been anticipating for so long. It can be a major challenge for family members to move past this difficult feeling, but it is necessary to do so, for emotional survival.

How do people manage to cope with major tragedies in their lives without being consumed by rage or despair? A full exploration of this important topic is beyond the scope of this book. Suffice it to say that most individuals are able to master a difficult challenge when it befalls them, somehow relying on the considerable adaptive abilities that they have developed in life. For many, religion is a great source of comfort. Those who feel that any terrible adversity they are forced to experience in this life will be rewarded in the afterlife are able to endure terrible degrees of hardship with this belief as a source of solace. Others manage in different ways. However, there are some who are unable to move past the misery, and they become laden with despair, rage, or both.

One of the most important tenets that family members must keep in mind in coping with Alzheimer's disease is to be angry at the *disease*, and not the *person* with the disease. This is easier said than done, of course, particularly when certain behaviors that are brought about by the illness can be quite irritating. Furthermore, it is normal to want to have a concrete object or person at which to direct one's rage, not an abstract, invisible enemy such as Alzheimer's. As discussed in the previous chapter, some will displace their anger onto other people, such as the doctor who coldly made the diagnosis of Alzheimer's disease and walked away, as in Mel and Gloria's case. Others might displace their anger onto an event, such as the painful divorce of an adult child or a legal entanglement with an unpleasant neighbor, and feel that the traumatic event "caused" the disease. While it may be that significant stressors such as these might hasten the appearance of Alzheimer's, they certainly do not cause the illness. In all such cases, the disease was developing, anyway, but may not yet have reached sufficient severity to be recognized. Nevertheless, there is a natural human tendency to try to find an explanation for terrible things that happen, to try to find someone, or something, to blame. Perhaps it is better to be irate with the litigious neighbor for "causing" the illness, rather than expressing anger at the disease victim, which almost always makes the situation worse. But blaming anyone or anything other than the disease itself does not help the family member move past these difficult emotions toward fully facing and experiencing the profound feelings of grief that lie at the center of the family care partner's emotional journey.

Some family members, when confronted about their anger, will be quite uncomfortable thinking of themselves as harboring such a feeling and will stress that it is not anger that they feel, but merely irritation, annoyance, frustration, or some other description that carries a less severe connotation to them than anger. Probably this represents the defense of minimization, and it does no good to insist that it really is anger that he is feeling. Whatever one chooses to call the feeling, it is more useful to explore how pervasive the feeling is; toward what it is directed, exactly; how it affects the family member; and how it ultimately expresses itself, because it nearly always does.

Once again, it is worth emphasizing that these feelings of anger are extremely common, to the point where one should view them as normal reactions to very difficult circumstances, unless they become very pervasive or get acted out in ways that are destructive to the person with the disease. Nevertheless, the anger still needs to be understood in order for the family member to move forward emotionally. Most family members seem able to do this, fortunately.

However, some family members find themselves preoccupied

with resentment toward the person with the disease. They may not allow this to come to the surface very often, but it may nevertheless color their day-to-day interactions with him. There may be less warmth, less closeness, less empathy, less pleasure in interacting with him, and less desire to spend time with him. Anger may not be expressed with wrathful outpourings (although those can certainly occur), but in other ways, such as neglecting the needs of the person with the disease or with subtle or not-so-subtle belittling, sarcasm, or criticism. These understated expressions of anger can be more destructive than the occasional angry outburst. They are sufficiently understated so that the impaired individual may not fully realize that he is being criticized but merely ends up feeling worse about himself. This type of restrained expression of hostility can continue for a very long time, and it poisons the relationship between the family member and the person with the disease. The family member himself may not be aware of the anger or destructiveness of his approach.

Some feel that the act of expressing one's anger is somehow good for the individual who feels it, that expressing one's anger leads to feeling less anger. Generally, however, venting anger usually does not reduce the amount of anger felt; both the expresser and the victim come away from the interaction with different but often equally negative feelings. The solution to the anger problem is not to learn how to express it effectively or to learn how to suppress it, but to examine why it is being felt so strongly in the first place.

....

Victor and Annabelle had been married for twenty-three years. Both had previous marriages that ended in divorce. While Annabelle's two daughters from her first marriage stayed involved in her life, Victor's three children from his first marriage rarely saw or spoke to him. Victor and Annabelle did not have children together.

The relationship was a less than perfect one. Victor had been successful in business and was generous with money, but he spent a great deal of time with his friends after work or playing golf on weekends. Annabelle would complain about their not spending much time together, but Victor seemed unsympathetic to her complaints. She considered taking up golf, but Victor indicated that he would not play with her if she did, because she was unlikely to reach his level of play. She gave up the idea. Victor was frequently critical of Annabelle. Whether it was her housekeeping, her appearance (she gradually put on about fifteen pounds during the course of the marriage), the lifestyle of her lesbian daughter, or her cooking, Victor always seemed to convey to her that she did not measure up to his standards. There was actually very little fighting; Victor was articulate and persistent about his point of view, and Annabelle felt she could never prevail. Instead, she focused her energies on trying to improve herself. If asked, both would have said they had a reasonably good marriage.

At sixty-eight, Victor was diagnosed with Alzheimer's disease. He did not accept this with grace and felt the doctors were wrong. But soon after getting diagnosed, Victor got terribly lost driving home from a golf outing two hours away. While he was driving around, trying to find his way, the car ran out of gas. Victor abandoned it and wandered aimlessly until the police spotted him. By then it was raining, hard. He told the policeman that his car had broken down (he did not realize it was simply out of gas) but could not direct the officer to it. Fortunately, another policeman came upon the abandoned car on the sidewalk of a side street and arranged to have it towed to the police station. Victor was brought to the police station also but was not allowed to take his car. Annabelle was called and was asked to come to get him and bring someone who could drive Victor's car home.

Annabelle's anxiety over Victor's not returning home when he was expected turned quickly to rage over the inconvenience and embarrassment his "carelessness" (as she saw it) was causing her. Rather than attributing this behavior to his Alzheimer's disease, she assumed he had been out drinking with his golf buddies and it was inebriation, not dementia, that caused all of this to happen. She felt this way despite the fact that the police had said nothing about alcohol, just that he seemed too confused to drive himself home safely. Annabelle fumed all the way to the police station, some forty-five minutes away. Finally, her daughter Claudia, whom she had brought along to drive Victor's car home, suggested that maybe it wasn't alcohol at all, but his recently diagnosed Alzheimer's, that caused the problem. Annabelle seemed surprised at that revelation and agreed that it might be so, but this didn't seem to lessen her anger very much.

When they got to the police station, Victor was told that he could not drive the car home, as they had also taken his driver's license and were sending it to the department of motor vehicles. He would need to undergo a written driving test and an on-the-road examination in order to regain his license. Claudia drove Victor's car to her house, which enraged and humiliated him.

Victor was exhausted and relatively quiet on the way home. But the next morning, he insisted on going over to Claudia's to get his car and stated that he planned to drive himself to the DMV to take the tests. He did not understand that he was not permitted to do this, nor could he understand the need to wait until he was officially notified by the DMV, as the police had explained to him. He would certainly not consider that the events of the day before might mean he should give up driving for good. In fact, he was already forgetting most of the details. All of this infuriated Annabelle still further. She reminded him, angrily, that the doctor had said he had Alzheimer's disease, and she told him that he probably had no business being on the road at all.

....

What made Annabelle so angry? Perhaps she was simply very annoyed at the inconvenience of having to pick up her daughter and drive in the rain to fetch her husband. In addition, she was embarrassed and humiliated by having to pick him up at a police station. Certainly Victor's denial and forgetfulness the next day, and his unreasonable demands about driving himself to the DMV were trying. But Annabelle's anger seemed too extreme to be explained completely by these factors. In addition, her anger seemed to override any concern for Victor's well-being through all of this and also pushed aside any worries she might have had about the confusion that led to the driving incident in the first place.

Annabelle persisted in feeling irate toward Victor. She finally went to see Victor's doctor, alone, to ask what could be done to "force" Victor to recognize and accept his disease. But it quickly became clear that the more immediate issue was for her to understand the sources of her own rage and to learn how to cope more effectively with it. She initially did not understand why she felt so much anger and did not know what she could do to lessen it. But she did acknowledge that it made her quite distressed to feel such strongly negative feelings toward someone whom she had loved for many years. Initially, she was quite resistant to examining her anger, feeling that it was an emotion "anyone" would feel after having gone through what she had just experienced with Victor. However, after much discussion, it became clear that the car incident had unleashed a wellspring of irate feelings that Annabelle had been keeping inside of her, probably for years. While Annabelle appeared to passively accept Victor's criticisms and inattentiveness over the years, she had in fact been building feelings of resentment for a long time. She had kept this hidden, even from herself to a great degree, and felt that being taken care of by Victor as she aged was an acceptable trade-off. But with his diagnosis, and now this event, it became clear that it was *she* who would be taking care of *him*, not the other way around. All of her passive acceptance of his mistreatment of her over the years was for naught, and with that awareness, her anger had boiled to the surface. Eventually, she started psychotherapy with a local professional to help her come to terms with her feelings about the situation.

Annabelle's wrath served another purpose, as well. By focusing so exclusively on how furious she felt toward Victor, she was able to avoid facing the frightening realities of his illness and the loss of someone upon whom she had depended for so long. In this sense, her rage also served a defensive purpose, by pushing aside those more frightening thoughts about losing him to the illness. On some level, it was easier for her to feel anger than to feel frightened and abandoned. It should be obvious that the "choice" to feel angry, rather than to feel abandoned, is certainly not a conscious one. It would seem that a self-protective part of her mind automatically, and outside of the conscious realm, made a substitution that seemed to be more acceptable, at least in the short run. Working productively with these feelings, alone or with the help of a confidante or therapist, however, involves bringing this process into consciousness, so that the underlying feelings, as difficult as they are, can be confronted, explored, felt, and eventually mastered.

In Alzheimer's disease, perhaps more than in most illnesses, unresolved family dynamics, perhaps long buried or ignored, will return with a vengeance. As more than one angry family member has said, "the chickens come home to roost" in this illness. It may be, for example, a matter of unresolved resentments in a marriage that come to the fore again (or for the first time), as in the case of Annabelle and Victor; or it may be a conflicted parent-child relationship that gets replayed, with a formerly domineering and frightening parent now brought to heel for the first time because of the disease.

Other dynamics, as well, can lead to excessive anger among family members.

....

Allen and Rebecca had been married for forty-two years. They had no children. They had gotten along reasonably well over the years. Rebecca was a successful bookkeeper prior to her retirement. Allen was a painter, talented but never commercially very successful. They lived reasonably comfortably, primarily on her income. Allen was gregarious, always needing to be the center of attention, and Rebecca was comfortable playing her assigned role in the background. They had lots of acquaintances but few close friends as a couple. Rebecca was extremely close to her sister, Ruth, who lived quite nearby. They would talk on the phone at least daily and would see each other frequently for lunch. Their husbands were not very fond of each other, so they rarely socialized as couples. This disappointed Rebecca, but as long as she was able to maintain her close individual connection to Ruth, she did not make an issue of it.

Rebecca began to show signs of Alzheimer's disease around age seventy-two, about two years after she retired. She became repetitive, less attentive to keeping the house tidy, and eventually began to have trouble managing the household bills and checkbook, as she had always done. Allen did not seem very aware of these growing difficulties until Ruth called him to express her concerns about Rebecca's growing difficulties. As a result of the phone call, Allen began to notice her increasing problems with performing her daily tasks. Allen seemed rather unsympathetic toward these matters. He felt irritated that Rebecca's increasing needs necessitated his spending more time managing household tasks instead of working on his painting. In the midst of all of these concerns, Allen had received a commission for a series of illustrations, and he was worried that he would not be able to concentrate fully on his work and complete it on schedule because of all the added chores for which he was now responsible. He became increasingly angry with Rebecca for the imposition her illness was causing him, and on more than one occasion told her, in a rage, that she should go to live with her sister, or go to a nursing home. It was as if the most important consequence of her developing this devastating disease was the impact it was having and would continue to have on his professional life, and it made him deeply furious with her for "doing this" to him.

Allen's self-involvement had not caused a major upheaval in their relationship until now, because Rebecca had always felt that it was acceptable to play the role of the supportive wife to what she felt was her "more important" husband-artist, and she busied herself in and derived a great deal of satisfaction from her work. She wrote off much of his selfishness over the years to his "artistic temperament" and seemed very content to care for him and manage the mundane details of their marriage. She had, in fact, taken no small degree of pride in seeing herself as the supportive spouse whose travails permitted her artistic spouse to pursue his creative life. Allen, of course, was quite satisfied with this arrangement, as well, until Rebecca's developing illness forced him to become more involved in the household and, especially, in meeting her needs.

Shame

Each of the emotions discussed up to this point—anxiety, guilt, and anger—primarily have to do with the family member's relationship with the person with Alzheimer's disease. Shame, however, brings the outside world into the life of the person with the disease and the family member. Shame is only experienced in the presence of others. That presence may be real, or it may be what the family member imagines about how others will react. Real or abstract, there is at least one additional person who is observing the situation and (in the mind of the family member) making negative judgments of some kind.

Other emotions closely related to shame are embarrassment, humiliation, disgrace, and mortification. There may be subtle differences in the meaning or interpretation of these terms, although here they are considered synonyms. However, as with anger, family members may deny a particular feeling, only to acknowledge one that is essentially synonymous but that seems to them to have connotations that are less severe, more socially acceptable, or more dignified. For example, someone may deny feeling disgraced by their loved one's behavior, but will admit to a degree of embarrassment. A family member might balk at the notion of feeling ashamed of a loved one who behaved inappropriately in a public setting but will admit to finding the incident somewhat mortifying. Whatever words are used to describe his emotional response to the inappropriate behavior, it can be very useful for the family member to explore his own reactions to the situation—why did the behavior of the person with Alzheimer's cause such a reaction in him, in the first place? After all, one is not responsible for the behaviors of a person with Alzheimer's, but family members often react that way.

What behaviors lead to feelings of shame? In addition to memory loss or confusion, observable to others, behaviors that are socially unpleasant, such as bowel or bladder incontinence, are a common source of shame. So are poor manners or sloppy eating behaviors in a restaurant. Talking out loud in church or a theater or another setting where quiet is expected is another. Behaviors that are secondary to disinhibited behavior, which so commonly occurs in Alzheimer's, are a common cause of shame. In short, anything that the person with Alzheimer's does which indicates to others that she is not able or willing to fully control her own actions, or not able to conform with social expectations of propriety can lead to feelings of shame on the part of the family member.

The person with the disease may no longer be able to prevent such behaviors and may also have lost the mental capacity to experience feelings of shame or embarrassment, particularly as the disease worsens. Under those circumstances, it is especially important for family members to do whatever they can to protect the person's dignity, and to try, for his sake, to avoid situations that would be embarrassing or shameful to him, if he were still capable of experiencing such feelings.

....

Roger had always been an upstanding, well-respected, and well-liked member of his community. He was active in his church and at the weekly meetings of the Rotary Club. As his Alzheimer's developed, however, he became mildly disinhibited in a variety of respects. One of the earliest signs of disinhibition was that he would notice anyone who was slightly overweight and comment on this in full voice, wherever he was. While his family found this both surprising and somewhat amusing, they were also aware that before his illness, Roger would never make any comments that could be offensive or hurtful to others and that he would be mortified if he were aware he was doing something so socially inappropriate. When he began to make such comments at the parish house coffee hour after church services, his family quickly learned that they needed to keep him away from overweight individuals, since they could not get him to stop making such remarks (which they had tried, unsuccessfully, to do). When a large person would start to come his way, his family would turn him around and walk in the other direction to try to limit the chance of his embarrassing himself with other churchgoers, most of whom he had known, at least superficially, for many decades. When Roger commented one day, in a loud voice, that the new minister was "rather pudgy," the family finally decided that it was easiest simply to avoid these church gatherings altogether. They would tell him that the coffee hour after the service had been cancelled, or they needed to rush home immediately after the service, for some invented reason. They knew he would want to have his fellow churchgoers remember him as the gentleman he had been before his illness, and not as the socially inappropriate person he was becoming.

....

In this case, it is clear that Roger's family, whatever they personally felt about his behavior, wanted to preserve his reputation and his dignity, and they acted accordingly, since Roger was no longer able to keep from behaving in this way.

It is important to consider whether the shame is felt in behalf of the person with Alzheimer's disease, or in behalf of the family member herself—or both. Although it can be challenging to try to preserve the dignity of a person with Alzheimer's when he is no longer able to do so because of the illness, the most emotionally difficult situations arise when it is the family member's *own* sense of shame that becomes the issue. Although this may be quite common, family members are extremely reluctant to recognize that their loved one's behavior makes them feel ashamed. They are often quick to rationalize that "it's not his fault" and that, because they *shouldn't* feel ashamed, they believe they *don't* feel ashamed. But often, they do. Why should one feel personally ashamed because of the behavior of another? There is no logical reason, of course, but it often occurs because of what the family member feels the behavior says or implies about the family member, himself.

....

Peter and Gwen had been married for almost eight years before Peter developed Alzheimer's disease. Both had been married previously and had divorced. Peter was sixty-nine, and Gwen was fifty-four at the time of his diagnosis. With the onset of his illness, Gwen acknowledged that she felt somewhat "cheated," because of the relatively few healthy years they had been able to share, but she loved Peter and was a good care partner.

As his disease progressed, Peter began to develop some concerning disinhibited behaviors. Because Gwen was still working, she had hired a private care partner, Flora, to spend a few hours during the day with Peter. Peter was fond of Flora, and one afternoon, he propositioned her sexually. Flora joked it off, but when this happened a second time and included Peter's making some inappropriate comments about parts of her anatomy, Flora more forcefully told Peter to stop it, and reported this behavior to Gwen the next time she saw her. Gwen was extremely embarrassed and ashamed by this, and she furiously confronted Peter as soon as Flora left the house. Peter denied the accusation. It was never clear if he denied it in order to lessen Gwen's anger at him or because he simply did not recall the incidents.

When Peter made openly sexual comments to Flora a third time, about a week later, Flora decided that she did not wish to continue to work with him under these circumstances and gave notice that she was leaving. At this point, Gwen accepted Flora's resignation and asked the agency to send someone else as soon as possible. Gwen alternated between feeling ashamed of Peter's behavior and feeling (defensively) that the cause of the problem, in the first place, might have been Flora's provocative, tight clothing.

The agency sent Beverly, an older and somewhat obese and homely care partner, and things went well for several weeks. Gwen felt relieved that the problem seemed to be solved. However, at that point, Peter grabbed one of Beverly's breasts while she was serving him lunch and seemed unremorseful when Beverly told him, in no uncertain terms, that the behavior was unacceptable. Beverly told Gwen about the incident when she returned home later that afternoon, although it was clear she wasn't upset by it, perhaps more amused than anything else. However, Gwen was both deeply ashamed (perhaps even more so than when this happened with Flora) and furious with Peter for his behavior. She made an appointment to meet with Peter's doctor, alone, to discuss these behaviors and to find out if any medication might be helpful in controlling his impulses.

During the meeting with Peter's doctor, it became apparent how humiliated Gwen felt about these incidents. She had never thought of Peter as a lecherous person before, and although part of her knew that these behaviors were related to his disease, she was still deeply troubled by them.

The doctor asked her to describe the history of their relationship in more detail. Gwen indicated that she became involved with Peter after her divorce from her first husband but while Peter was still married. They carried on an affair secretly for about six months. She never felt that she destroyed his marriage, as it was clear from the time they met that Peter's own marriage was on the brink of dissolution; perhaps their affair had simply hurried that process along. She had never felt consciously guilty about her role in his divorce.

After they were married, Peter and Gwen continued to have an enjoyable physical relationship, although the frequency of their encounters declined gradually. Once Peter's Alzheimer's became manifest, Gwen found it initially difficult, and then impossible, to continue to have a sexual relationship with him, as she had come to feel more like a provider of care and less like a wife and sexual partner. Initially, Peter attempted to continue their intimacy, but this was met with gentle rebuffs from Gwen. Gradually, he seemed content with occasional hugging and cuddling, which Gwen strictly controlled and would quickly terminate whenever she determined that Peter was becoming desirous of something more.

In addition to her intellectual understanding that sexual inappropriateness not infrequently occurs in Alzheimer's disease, Gwen wondered if she had somehow provoked this behavior in Peter by her own unwillingness to continue her sexual relationship with him. She even wondered if he had originally become involved with her, years ago, because he was no longer sexually active with his first wife. She had, in fact, asked him this when they first were married, and he insisted that he had fallen in love with Gwen and that their sexual relationship had grown out of that, not the other way around. She had always believed his response, although she found herself wondering about that now. It became clear that this incident had reawakened long-buried guilt feelings about getting involved with a married man, and perhaps more recent guilt feelings of depriving Peter sexually at this difficult time in his life. In discussing all of this with Peter's doctor, Gwen came to realize that her deep sense of shame about what had happened with Flora and Beverly was because she felt that they would somehow blame her for this, and that they would somehow believe that Peter's sexual behavior was a result of Gwen's not fulfilling him sexually, just as she worried now that his involvement with her initially may have been, at least in part, because of his lack of sexual fulfillment with his first wife.

....

Gwen was only able to stop feeling so ashamed of Peter's behavior when she realized that she was ashamed for herself, more than for Peter. She needed to understand the possible roots of this shame in earlier decisions she had made in her life (for example, her involvement with Peter when he was still married) and to understand that she felt that Flora and Beverly—and by extension, perhaps, everyone else—would judge her as inadequate, withholding, and unsatisfying to Peter. As she came to realize that she felt this way, she also recognized how unrealistic her feelings were: the care partners were not judging her in any way; being experienced in the field, they had undoubtedly dealt with this kind of behavior before. She came to realize that Peter's behavior did not mean that she was an inadequate wife; his behavior said nothing whatsoever about her, but only about his disease. It also was useful for her to realize that she had some long-unresolved feelings about the beginnings of their relationship that she needed to consider further, but at this point she had to focus on how she could best care for Peter going forward. It was also very helpful to her to mention Peter's inappropriate sexual behavior at a support group meeting and hear from two other wives that their husbands had done the same thing.

Other types of disinhibited behaviors seem to be an exaggeration of prior personality traits and can thus also cause feelings of care partner shame.

....

Ethel had been widowed many years earlier, and when she developed Alzheimer's disease, she moved in with her daughter Marlene and Marlene's husband, Joel. Marlene and Ethel had always had a contentious relationship; Ethel had been critical of Marlene and often quite irritable with her, picking fights with her for no apparent reason. She seemed to favor Marlene's brother, Ben, while they were growing up, often comparing her unfavorably to him, in terms of their grades in school, popularity, athletic ability, or her rebelliousness. Ben was now married and lived in Ohio, and he came home rarely.

Marlene had some misgivings about having Ethel move in with them, but felt that it was the right thing to do. In addition, she hoped that by letting her mother move in to her home, Ethel might come to feel more loving toward her, stop criticizing her so much, and comparing her unfavorably to her brother.

Soon after Ethel moved in, Marlene realized how impaired her mother was; previously, she had been partially able to hide it behind a facade of bravado and her intimidating style. For a short time after moving in, Ethel seemed to lessen her criticisms of Marlene, perhaps because of her appreciation for the support she was receiving, but before long Ethel began again to be highly critical of Marlene for nearly everything. Although she previously spoke to her in a somewhat harsh or condescending tone, now, she raised her voice, so at times she literally screamed at her. Marlene found this upsetting, understandably, and discovered that if she tried to defend herself, it only made the screaming worse. Unfortunately, it continued when Marlene would take Ethel out shopping, or for lunch, and Marlene felt very ashamed to be yelled at by her mother in public. Not surprisingly, Ethel's yelling turned heads, and even though Marlene knew this was not her fault and that it was due to Ethel's personality, exacerbated by her illness, she would find herself blushing uncontrollably whenever it happened. Marlene assumed that others would notice the blushing and that it would confirm in the minds of observers that Marlene really was in the wrong about something and deserved the tongue-lashing she was receiving.

Marlene felt furious at her mother for the humiliation she was causing her and decided that she would no longer go to public places with her. Ethel continued to rant at her daughter frequently at home in a high volume. Marlene worried that the neighbors would hear and wonder what was wrong. She assumed they would blame her (Marlene) for upsetting the elderly and demented Ethel. The situation worsened when the warm weather came and windows were open. Marlene was sure her mother could be heard down the block. Finally, one of her neighbors (who was also a good friend) told Marlene that she shouldn't tolerate her mother yelling at her like that, and that Marlene should put her in a home if it continued. Marlene felt relieved that someone close to her understood the situation accurately. Eventually, Marlene did place her mother in assisted living when her care needs, along with the yelling, increased to the point where Marlene was becoming exhausted, depressed, and angry nearly all of the time. She realized that she had been unsuccessful in changing the dynamics of her relationship with her mother and continued to feel bad about that, but she was also quite relieved to have her go into a facility and become free of Ethel's daily unreasonable and unkind treatment of her.

....

When Marlene told this story to her mother's new doctor at the assisted living facility, the doctor told her that she had acted appropriately, first by no longer taking her out in public, and eventually by placing her when she did. It was also quite obvious that her deep sense of shame over her mother's behavior was in part a feeling of embarrassment for her mother (who seemed oblivious to what others might think) but even more so, it had to do with her feeling ashamed about what others would think of *her*, Marlene. Even though she recognized that it was unrealistic to think that people would assume she was the one in the wrong, she could not help but feel this way, or control her blushing when it happened. She related events from her childhood when her mother would scold her in public, including one incident when her mother actually slapped her in a department store when she was a young child. She vividly recalled the humiliation she had felt at that time. It seemed clear that Ethel's yelling might have greater poignancy because it recalled those early humiliations Marlene suffered.

Chapter Four

Understanding Grief in the Family Care Partner

The central emotional experience of the Alzheimer's family is grief over the gradual loss of the loved one, before actual physical death occurs (Noyes et al. 2010). Grieving for the loss of the person who is living with the disease begins very early in the illness and generally worsens throughout its course (Ott et al. 2007; Sanders et al. 2008).

This chapter reviews a number of common features of this distinctive type of grief; chapter 5 discusses the stages of grief in the Alzheimer's care partner.

Grief and Depression

While grief shares a number of similarities with depression, it is important to recognize that grief and depression are *not* the same. Grief is a normal human emotion, however painful it may be. Grief is the emotional response to the loss of someone or something that is held very dear. Usually, it is a person toward whom one feels a strong affection, but grief can also be felt over other losses — the death of a pet or the destruction of one's home in a fire or tornado, for example. Grief can also be felt in response to losing something more abstract, such as one's youth or one's physical health. This is an important aspect of grief in Alzheimer's, discussed below.

While grief is a normal human emotion, depression is not. Nor is depression the same as simple sadness. The term depression is used in a variety of ways. Sometimes, in common usage, for example, it is used to convey mild feelings of unhappiness or frustration, as in "I'm so depressed—I was going to play tennis today, and now it's raining!" Or the term might be used to describe simple feelings of sadness or disappointment, as in "I was depressed that I didn't get as good a grade on the test as I had hoped." However, in clinical terms, depression refers to an *abnormal* emotional state in which the individual feels a depth of sadness beyond what would be expected, or sometimes when there is no apparent precipitant whatsoever. Often, a host of other physical or psychological symptoms accompany depression. At times, particularly for the elderly in depressive states, the emotion of sadness is less prominent than other symptoms, such as fatigue, worry, somatic complaints, pessimism, irritability, or the loss of the ability to experience pleasure. There is often a great deal of self-criticism, or criticism of others, in states of depression, whereas that is not the case in pure grief. It is often said that in sadness or grief, the individual is unhappy with something that has occurred, while in depression the individual is unhappy with himself. While depression (if mild) might resolve on its own, more severe depression usually requires some form of treatment. On the other hand, working with grief so that the individual is able to move forward through the process of adaptation and, ultimately, to reach a state of acceptance usually does not require psychiatric treatment and is best addressed by the considerations described in this volume.

Despite the differences between grief and depression described above, it is very important to keep in mind that grief can, in fact, lead to a serious depressive episode. It is always important for the clinician to determine if the individual who has been in grief has now deteriorated into a state of depression. However, the distinction between grief and depression can be quite difficult to determine, at times. The final chapter, "Understanding and Coping with Stress in the Family Care Partner," reviews the differentiation between grief and depression in greater detail.

The Subjective Experience of Grief

How is grief experienced? John Bowlby, the British psychologist famed for his pioneering work on human attachment, has described it this way: "The loss of a loved person is one of the most intensely painful experiences any human can suffer" (Bowlby 1980). Although Bowlby was referring to grief that occurs after death, the protracted, chronic grief of the Alzheimer's family member causes similar anguish and is complicated by characteristics that are unique to the Alzheimer's situation. In fact, many family members who have also suffered the death of a loved one from an illness other than Alzheimer's have said that coping with the losses associated with Alzheimer's disease is a more difficult anguish to endure.

Although each person's experience of grief is unique, the following case illustrates a rather typical experience.

....

Sylvia and Dominick had been married for more than fifty years when Dominick began to show signs of Alzheimer's disease. Sylvia knew what to expect as the disease progressed: both Dominick's mother and older brother had suffered from the illness, and she and Dominick had been very involved in helping care for his mother during the last years of her life. Sylvia was determined to keep Dominick at home throughout the illness, and his passive manner and general good nature in the face of his illness helped to make this possible. Yet as the disease progressed, Dominick was less and less "present," and required increasing amounts of physical care. After several years, Sylvia became exhausted and decided that she needed to place Dominick in a local assisted living facility for a week of respite care, so that she could regain her strength, emotionally and physically. When reporting this very reasonable decision (which was nevertheless tinged with a great deal of guilt), Sylvia described Dominick's illness as increasingly difficult to endure. She found herself feeling sad almost all the time, and while Dominick presented no behavioral difficulties, assisting him with activities of daily living and constantly monitoring him to ensure his safety was wearing on her tremendously. She said that she loved Dominick more than ever, despite his illness, but that she was increasingly lonely, even though her children, who lived out of state, called frequently, and several neighbors would occasionally drop in for coffee or to play cards. Sylvia described her situation as "I'm alone but I'm not alone." She thought that the period of respite would help break up what felt like an increasingly difficult routine of caring for Dominick, taking care of her house, and overeating to try to cope with her sadness. She compared this difficult state of affairs to "a funeral without an end."

....

Grief is psychologically distinct from the emotions described in the preceding chapter—anxiety, guilt, anger, and shame—and it is also distinct from the various defense mechanisms discussed in chapter 3. However, the family member's defenses and at times the four emotions listed above are used, unconsciously, to deflect, lessen, or avoid the terrible anguish of grief. Only after the family member permits herself to fully experience and acknowledge her grief can genuine emotional healing begin to take place. Ever since the onset of the illness, of course, the successful care partner has been adjusting to the new realities of the person transformed by Alzheimer's, but a more fundamental adaptation can take place only after grief has been openly experienced and acknowledged. This more fundamental adaptation involves not only learning to react appropriately to changes in the behavior of the person with the illness; it also includes adapting to profound changes in the relationship between the person with the disease and the family member. When this is successful, it will permit the family care partner to move forward toward a state of acceptance, with equanimity.

Common Features of Care Partner Grief

There are several essential features of grief associated with Alzheimer's disease that are particularly common and that make an already anguishing situation even more difficult for the family member to endure. These features are compounded loss, anticipatory grief, ambiguous loss, disenfranchised grief, loss of a sense of shared reality, and loss of the hope for reconciliation.

Compounded Loss

The losses that occur in Alzheimer's disease are many, perhaps in contrast to the grief caused by the death of a loved one from another illness. The losses in Alzheimer's often occur one right after another, with little opportunity to process each one individually, thus creating what is called *compounded loss*. In this difficult situation, one loss cannot be accepted or resolved fully before the next occurs. Even relatively small events can trigger intense emotional reactions because of the impact of multiple losses occurring in a short time. Compounded loss is often experienced as the feeling of being burdened that comes with being unable to process and fully understand what is happening as it occurs. Even families who thoroughly educate themselves about the disease and the many changes that will occur can be overcome by the anguish of trying to handle so many losses over such a short period of time.

Anticipatory Grief

Anticipatory grief refers to the feelings of grief that individuals experience prior to the actual loss, by death, of a loved one (Lindemann 1944). Frequently, this concept is applied to the emotions of family members of people dying from cancer or other terminal medical conditions. It has been postulated that, by going through the stages of grief while the loved one is still alive, the grief at the actual time of death is less severe.

In Alzheimer's disease, the situation is somewhat different. While the family member may, in fact, feel grief in anticipation of the loved one's eventual death, much of the anguish of the Alzheimer's care partner is due to losses that have already occurred. As noted earlier, these losses are largely the intangible ones, such as losing the companionship of someone whose personality is now clouded by Alzheimer's, or losing the wit and problem-solving abilities that were so strongly valued throughout the relationship, or losing the opportunity for sexual intimacy.

While the term *anticipatory grief* is sometimes used in the literature to describe the anguish of the Alzheimer's family member prior to the disease victim's death, this is different, psychologically and emotionally, from the anticipatory grief of the family member whose loved one is dying from a physical, not cognitive, illness. In that situation, the individual generally remains very much present, cognitively and interpersonally, at least until very near the end. In the case of Alzheimer's, much of what is sometimes labeled as anticipatory grief is not really "anticipatory" at all. From the earliest stages of the disease, care partners frequently report "missing the person"; this is not something they anticipate with dread for the future, but something that is already very much a reality. Of course, there may well be elements of true anticipatory grief present as well, as loved ones anticipate that the disease will worsen and that, for example, an afflicted spouse who now recognizes him will at some point in the future no longer be able to do so. And there is, also, the sad anticipation of death, at some point in the future (Garand 2012).

Does the grief felt by the Alzheimer's family member during the disease victim's life ease the grieving that he will experience when the loved one actually dies? In some cases, that would seem to be true, but many family members describe a new, overwhelming wave of grief that comes at the time of actual death. Perhaps it is the final, inescapable reality that death brings; it may also be that the countless moments of grief that were felt with each episode of clinical worsening are reexperienced when the individual actually dies. In any case, family members are often surprised at how much anguish they feel at the time of death, even as they also experience a sense of relief that the suffering has finally come to an end.

....

Claire and Irving were married for more than forty years when Irving began to show signs of Alzheimer's. Theirs was an extremely close and happy relationship, and the reality of the illness hit Claire very hard. Early on, both she and Irving were filled with denial, but as time (and symptoms) went on, she began to recognize, with growing sadness, that the disease was transforming him profoundly.

When Irving gave up driving, Claire recognized this as a result of his clinical worsening, and she seemed even more upset with it than he was. They lived in a continuing care retirement community, where Irving had been quite active in a number of activities, and on several committees, but as his disease progressed, he was forced to give up his committee work, as he was not able to keep track of what was occurring. Gradually, he also had to stop playing bridge and singing in the chorale. He had been an avid reader of newspapers—a self-described "political junkie"—but he lost his ability to read the paper, even the headlines, although would often sit with the *New York Times* on his lap for the entire day, saying, when asked, that he was reading it. As Irving became less aware of world and national events, he was unable to name the candidates in the most recent presidential election or to name the new president. Claire greatly missed being able to talk with him about world news and politics, something they had done nearly every day, for decades, and she grieved deeply for that vital part of Irving that had been taken away by Alzheimer's. Eventually, he moved to the memory care unit, where he seemed content, although inactive and uninvolved in the daily life of the unit. Claire visited him daily, initially trying to engage him in conversation or an activity, with little success. Gradually, their time together consisted of sitting on the couch in the dayroom while Irving often dozed, or they would sit together in silence in the dayroom, holding hands, watching others in the unit. After about eight months in the memory care unit, Irving fell and fractured his hip. He was admitted to the nursing unit for palliative care but died after several days, from a massive pulmonary embolus.

Claire grieved at each new milestone in his illness: the termination of his driving; the loss of his ability to participate in the affairs of the facility; his inability to follow and talk about the news; and finally, his move out of their apartment to the memory care unit. By the time of his demise, Irving seemed to have minimal quality of life: he could not manage any of his activities of daily living independently; could not actively participate in any activities; spoke little, and often nonsensically, and frequently did not seem to recognize Claire. She had come to feel that his life was no longer meaningful to him in any way, and believed that death would be a blessing. But at the time of his passing, she was overwhelmed with a sense of loss once again.

....

As the situation with Claire and Irving illustrates, episodes of grief frequently occur at each step in the progression of the illness. While the loved one may, like Claire, feel that death would be a blessing, it still causes deep anguish when it finally occurs. It is probably impossible (and unnecessary) to determine how much of the family member's grief is "anticipatory"—thinking ahead about how the situation is going to worsen and end in death—and how much is grief over the very real losses that are occurring in the present and throughout the illness; both certainly lead to the anguish felt by the family member.

Ambiguous Loss

Ambiguous loss is a term coined by psychologist Pauline Boss to refer to an interpersonal loss that does not have a normal sense of closure (Boss 1999). According to Boss, there are two types of ambiguous loss. In the first, the individual is physically absent but remains psychologically present. This has been described as "Leaving without saying goodbye." Examples include prisoners of war or those missing in action, victims of disasters such as September 11 or Malaysia Airlines Flight 370, or even the absence of a parent as a result of divorce.

In the second type of ambiguous loss, the individual remains physically present, but is psychologically absent—or as Boss has described it, "The goodbye without leaving." This type of ambiguous loss occurs in a variety of conditions, and prominently in Alzheimer's disease. It is very difficult for the loved one to grieve for someone who may no longer be psychologically present as a spouse, a parent, a companion, or other intimate, but who remains very much present, physically, with ever-increasing needs for care that must be met. The very ambiguity of the relationship makes it challenging for the family member to acknowledge the loss, grieve, and move forward. Since the person with the disease usually changes so gradually, it is not possible for the family member to determine a specific point at which the loved one ceased to exist as he once was. Ambiguous loss—a loss that resists resolution and complicates the grieving process—is the result.

....

Hugh had Alzheimer's for more than seven years. When his wife, Daphne, suddenly died of a heart attack two years ago, Hugh moved in with his daughter, Karen, and her family. Karen did not work outside of the home, and now that her own children were in college, she was able to devote a great deal of her time to caring for Hugh, who was in the moderate stage of disease and needed a great deal of assistance with his activities of daily living. Karen had always been very close to her parents and was glad to be available for her father now. At one of Hugh's routine visits to monitor his dementia, Karen was asked how she (the care partner) was managing. She began to weep and indicated that, as her father's illness progressed, he had increasing difficulties with communication, significant apathy, and seemed less and less the man she had always known and idolized for his wit, his warmth, and his loving attention to his family. Karen's mother's death, two years earlier, had been a great shock and a tremendous sadness for her, but Karen felt that at least it was definitive—she was there one day, and gone the next. She reported that dealing with her father's slow demise—his gradual fading away as the person she loved, while needing more and more care every day—seemed like a much greater burden to her.

....

Karen's grief over her father's illness could not be fully resolved while he remained alive, at least physically, and while she was so involved in his daily care. She became frozen in a state of ambiguous loss. It was only after Hugh's actual death, about eighteen months later, that Karen was able to fully grieve for him and begin to move forward in her own life.

Disenfranchised Grief

The term *disenfranchised grief* refers to grief that is not publicly acknowledged or sanctioned (Doka 2002). This can occur in a variety of situations. For example, when a long-standing extramarital affair ends, there is usually little, if any, opportunity for those involved to speak openly about their feelings regarding the loss, because of the social stigma associated with having such a relationship in the first place. Another example is the loss of a beloved pet. Those who have never owned a pet will likely not understand or be able to fully sympathize with the anguish one might feel about such a loss. Disenfranchised grief can also occur in the parents of adult children with mental illness, criminality, alcoholism, or other substance abuse. It can also take place following a miscarriage or a terminated pregnancy.

In the case of Alzheimer's disease, the family member grieves for those aspects or qualities of the person that have been lost to the illness, as discussed above in regard to anticipatory grief. As noted, these elements of grief are not truly "anticipatory," in that the losses have already occurred. These losses may not be fully understood by those who have not had a similar experience of losing a loved one gradually to Alzheimer's disease. No matter how close or how caring one's friends may be, the ability to truly empathize with the anguish of the Alzheimer's care partner is limited in those who have not dealt personally with the disease.

Being able to genuinely process Alzheimer's grief and to move forward toward adaptation and, ultimately, acceptance is greatly facilitated by being able to share the experience with others who are, or have been, in the same situation. This is why it is so important for the Alzheimer's family member to connect with others in the Alzheimer's community. This critical matter is discussed in detail in chapter 7.

The grief of the Alzheimer's care partner is referred to as "disenfranchised" when he has been unable to have a full empathic exchange with someone who is or has been an Alzheimer's care partner. Without this experience, his grief feels misunderstood, or incompletely understood, and may even feel illegitimate. If others don't understand or are unable to identify with the grief of the care partner, he may even wonder if the feelings are valid—if he is "supposed to" feel this way or not. This can lead to a feeling of reluctance to express one's grief to others who are not current or former care partners.

....

Angelo and Theresa had been married for more than fifty years when Angelo began to show signs of Alzheimer's disease. Theresa struggled with accepting the diagnosis and then with the many tasks of providing care that fell to her. She was determined to keep Angelo at home rather than to place him in a nursing home, where his mother had languished, also with Alzheimer's, for the last several years of her life. Theresa was reluctant to attend a support group or ask for assistance from others. One

Saturday evening in late fall, Angelo left the house on foot unexpectedly and quickly disappeared before Theresa was even aware that he was no longer there. She got in the car and searched for him for forty-five minutes before finding him, just a few blocks away, cold and very confused. He stated that he was looking for a mailbox to mail a letter to his sister, who had died more than ten years earlier. He had written no such letter and in fact was no longer able to write at all. Theresa brought him home and gave him cocoa and a blanket. Fortunately, he was not harmed by his exposure to the elements.

The next morning, after church, Angelo and Theresa attended coffee hour at the parish house. Angelo, who no longer remembered the incident of wandering, seemed to be in good spirits and engaged in conversation with several of his old friends. Theresa was still shaken by what had occurred, and she told Leslie, one of her closest friends, about the incident. Leslie listened to the story, expressed some sympathy for Theresa's worry, and stated she was glad that Angelo was unharmed. She then told Theresa that she was lucky to still have a husband, since she (Leslie) and so many of their mutual friends had already been widowed. While Theresa understood the comment and realized that Leslie was only trying to cheer her up, she also realized from the interchange that Leslie had only a limited understanding of what she was going through as a care partner. Previously, whenever anyone had asked her about how the situation was going, Theresa would always reply that Angelo was doing well and was in good health, even though she realized as she said it that she was glossing over the grim realities of the situation. She now understood why. People—even her closest friends who cared deeply for her—could not really appreciate what she was experiencing with Angelo. She had no desire to explain it to them, for fear that they would see her as excessively complaining or not up to the challenges of providing care. Or, she worried they would tell her that she needed to place him in a nursing home. Perhaps they simply would not fully understand, which would leave her feeling frustrated, guilty, and diminished. She felt disenfranchised in her grief.

Loss of a Sense of Shared Reality

Although Alzheimer's is more than a memory disorder, the loss of memory creates much of the profound anguish in the sufferer and his family. Memory is the building block of one's personal narrative or autobiography and serves as a vital link in one's connections to others.

Couples and families build an ever-growing storehouse of shared experiences and memories over time, and these elements of "shared reality" become some of the most valued treasures in the relationship. This storehouse includes not only memories of shared events and activities, but also includes less tangible elements, such as personality characteristics and traits, and patterns of interaction between family members.

Beth had always relied on her husband Bert's high intelligence. She counted on him for guidance in everyday matters and felt comfortable assuming a more passive role. Bert was always the one in the family who "took care of things." When he was first diagnosed with Alzheimer's, Beth resisted acknowledging to herself the changes in his personality and abilities. One day her daughter said to her, "Mom, you take it personally that Dad is not as smart as he used to be." Beth realized that her daughter was correct: by denying what was happening to Bert, she had been attempting to maintain her view of him as the one who "took care of things" despite his gradually becoming capable of taking care of less and less. As she reflected on her daughter's comment, she realized that she now had to take a more active part in decision making for both herself and for Bert, and she was frightened by this. She grieved for the loss of this important element of their shared reality: her ability to count on Bert to "take care of things" and to take care of her at the same time.

....

Another common example of the loss of a shared reality owing to the disease is the spouse who has always taken pride in being a fine cook and serving her family nourishing, delicious meals, while her family highly valued her culinary expertise and appreciated being cared for in this way. As the disease develops, however, cooking ability generally declines, and the capacity to put together a meal of any kind usually becomes quite limited.

Other shared realities in the family—particularly those based on more remote memories or experiences—may remain until later in the disease. In the earlier stages of Alzheimer's, a family member may bring up these shared memories in an attempt to maintain a sense of connection with the individual who is becoming gradually more disconnected. Thus, photo albums from years ago will be brought out for frequent review, and "remember when" stories will often be told in an effort to maintain, or reawaken, the fading connection. Sadly, these remote memories eventually will be lost, and those treasured elements from the storehouse of shared reality will be gone. This can lead to some of the most profound feelings of loss and grief in the Alzheimer's situation. Even basic identities and relationships can eventually be blurred or completely lost by the illness. An example is the husband who believes that his wife is actually his mother, or his son is his brother. Even worse is the husband who no longer recognizes his wife or son as familiar at all.

....

George and Wilma and their twin children, Edwin and Elizabeth, spent a week or two every July at a cabin on a large lake about two hours north of their home. They began going there when the twins were six and returned every year until they completed high school. Every member of the family had fond memories of their time at the lake. The twins remembered sunburns, fireworks, going to the drive-in movie nearby, and having their first romances there. George and Wilma remembered teaching the twins how to swim and ride bicycles, fishing, and going to local flea markets and antique shops, among many other happy memories.

As George began to develop cognitive problems, Wilma and the twins would often talk about their summers at the lake with George, as he seemed to enjoy reminiscing. However, as George's illness progressed, he began to lose vital memories from the more remote past. One day, when George had progressed into the moderately severe stages of disease, Elizabeth brought up summer vacations at the lake. To her surprise and dismay, George had no recollection of those vacations whatsoever; he seemed to have lost all of his memories of their many happy times there. As Elizabeth brought up a number of events from those days, hoping to reawaken George's memory, he said that he possibly could have been there, a long time ago, with his first wife. In fact, George had never been married to anyone other than Wilma. Elizabeth felt deeply saddened that this treasured part of their family's history—their shared reality—had vanished completely from George's mind. She was saddened not only for him, but also for herself. She could no longer happily reminisce with him about those days and feel close to the father he had been before Alzheimer's.

Loss of the Hope for Reconciliation

While Alzheimer's may offer the opportunity (if not the imperative) to improve the quality of the relationship between the care partner and the person with the disease, there is a finite window of opportunity to do this, before the person with the illness becomes too cognitively impaired to participate meaningfully in such a rapprochement. This window of opportunity can close suddenly or unexpectedly, depending on the course of the illness. It may also close more gradually, but the family member may delay his attempt to reach a rapprochement until the disease has progressed too far to make such a resolution possible. Thus, the loss of the hope of reconciliation can occur when there is a conflicted relationship between a family member and an ill person, if the opportunity for attempting reconciliation has been missed.

....

Clara, an only child, was the primary care partner for her elderly mother Roxanne, who suffered from dementia. Clara believed her mother had never wanted her or loved her. As Roxanne's dementia advanced, she became increasingly agitated by Clara's attempts to help her. At times Roxanne expressed open animosity and even physical aggression. Clara obtained help from others, but she remained Roxanne's primary care partner. When asked to explain her willingness to care for her mother despite Roxanne's extreme behavior, Clara responded that all she had ever wanted was for her mother to affirm that she was a good daughter and that she loved her. "Now that she has dementia," she said, "I'm afraid I will never hear that."

....

At times, relationships are so steeped in negative feelings that no reconciliation will be possible.

....

David had been emotionally controlling, dominating, and sometimes an abusive husband to his wife, Susan, which led to a deeply ingrained pattern of treating one another with animosity and blame. David's Alzheimer's diagnosis did not change this pattern. Susan stayed angry and believed David was responsible for the changes in his personality and behavior. When it was brought to her attention that David had a brain disease that caused him to act in ways that were irrational or impulsive, she replied that he had always been a difficult person. When it was suggested she try to accept the reality of the disease and make her husband feel as safe and peaceful as possible, she was stunned. "He has always been mean," she asserted weakly.

....

In this case, Susan had little hope for reconciliation; in fact, she seemed to view her husband's illness-related behavior as simply a continuation of the hurts he had inflicted on her during the course of their marriage.

If there are unresolved issues in one partner who feels victimized by the relationship, he may be unable to muster the compassion and tremendous effort that a person with Alzheimer's disease requires. This is certainly one of the reasons why it is so important to attempt to reconcile a difficult relationship before it is too late.

Facing the Illness Openly

One of the important steps that will help the family member come to terms with her own grief about the illness is being able to talk openly with the afflicted person about the disease. The importance of breaking through the "conspiracy of silence" with the disease victim has been emphasized previously. While it may initially be difficult and upsetting for both parties, it is far better, in the long run, to openly face the unhappy realities of the situation.

....

Barbara's husband Charles was in the early stages of Alzheimer's disease. Barbara attended a family workshop with her adult children. The discussion concerned whether or not to talk about the disease with the loved one, and how to tell if he could still grasp the nature of the disease. Barbara mentioned that recently she was talking about the day's events with her husband in bed, when he both stated and asked at the same time if there was something wrong with him. Barbara, struggling with her own fear of what was happening to Charles, told him everything was okay.

....

Should Barbara have told Charles the truth about his illness? Had she missed an opportunity to connect with him? Perhaps. Barbara indicated that she was afraid of provoking fear in Charles, yet now she felt that she had abandoned him by not telling him the truth. While the fear of talking about the illness is both common and very understandable, there is no evidence that doing so causes harm to the disease victim (Lee et al. 2014). In fact, it may be a relief to the afflicted person to be able to talk openly about what she has sensed, or feared, about her cognitive functioning. It is almost always the case that what is feared but kept hidden seems much worse than whatever the reality might be.

Of course, when the person with Alzheimer's is highly motivated to hide or minimize her deficits, or is completely unaware of them, talking openly about the disease and its symptoms is certainly more difficult, but it is usually not impossible. In fact, it may even be *more* important to talk about it when there is a significant amount of fear and resistance. In chapter 2, denial and other elements of discordance between the person with the illness and the family member were discussed, and various approaches to addressing this problem were considered. These will not be reiterated here. However, when it seems impossible to have an open discussion about the illness, it is important to carefully consider whether it is the person with the disease or the family member himself who is more reluctant to discuss it. When the person with the disease is able to talk about her illness and her feelings about the changes that are occurring, this will often help the family member face his own feelings of loss and grief.

Chapter Five

Stages of Grief in the Family Care Partner

Grief in the Alzheimer's family member is at the center of his reaction to losing a loved one with this disease (Frank 2008). Feelings of grief begin with the earliest signs of the illness—often before a formal diagnosis has been made—and continue, usually with increasing intensity, as the disease progresses, with new feelings of loss occurring after physical death occurs (Schultz et al. 2008). It can be helpful in understanding this grief to conceptualize it as occurring in several stages: anguish, adaptation, and acceptance.

These stages often overlap, since the losses that occur do not happen all at the same time or in a simple, organized fashion. For example, a spouse may be reaching the final stage of grief, acceptance: he is beginning to genuinely accept, with equanimity, that his loved one no longer remembers the names or identities of their children. But as the disease progresses, the afflicted spouse gradually loses the ability to recognize her husband as well, and he reacts to this loss with a renewed sense of anguish. Adjusting to the anguish of this change will be the primary task of the second stage of grief, adaptation. In the third stage of grief, acceptance, the care partner is gradually able to come to terms with this new reality, with—it is to be hoped—a degree of equanimity rather than bitterness, anger, or despair. It is only then that the care partner can truly begin to move forward with his own life.

Anguish

The first stage of grief is called *anguish*. This describes the intense emotional distress caused by the care partner's full realization of loss. It is the initial feeling the family member experiences as she moves beyond defensiveness and past the various emotions discussed in chapter 3. In this stage, she faces, in many respects for the first time, the profound losses associated with the realization of having a loved one with Alzheimer's disease. Because of this anguish, there may be an attempt to return to the emotional protection of the defenses. However, by this point, the powerful realities of the current situation will likely defeat any attempts the care partner may attempt at defensive avoidance.

In addition to experiencing the pain of these losses, the care partner will usually review the relationship she had with the afflicted individual, prior to the illness. Part of her anguish comes from the awareness that her relationship with the loved one has now changed, forever.

....

Aaron and Stephanie had been married for nine years. Both had been previously married and divorced; Stephanie is fourteen years younger than Aaron. Their relationship had been a very good one. Both had been in unhappy marriages previously, and despite their significant age difference, they felt that they had finally found "soul mates" when they first got together. They shared many common interests, including hiking, tennis, and listening to jazz.

Unfortunately, after just eight years of marriage, Aaron began to show signs of cognitive decline. He had recently retired, and both he and Stephanie attributed his inability to keep track of the date and other common matters to the fact that he was no longer going to work and needing to remember such things. However, as time passed, Aaron's memory difficulties increased, and he seemed unable or uninterested to pursue many of his previous activities. Stephanie encouraged him onto the tennis court regularly, but his game became erratic, and he was completely unable to keep score. On one occasion, he hit a serve that was out of bounds, and when Stephanie called it as such, he lost his temper, cursed loudly at her, and stormed off the court. This was very uncharacteristic for him and obviously quite upsetting and embarrassing for her.

Although Aaron's doctor had indicated that Aaron had some form of memory disorder and had prescribed anti-dementia medication (which he took for a few weeks only, then stopped), this event led them to see the specialist who had been previously recommended. The specialist confirmed the diagnosis of Alzheimer's disease. This seemed to eliminate any remaining denial that Stephanie, at least, had about his condition, and she felt devastated—anguished—for Aaron, and for herself.

Although she tried to hide the intensity of her feelings from Aaron, who still harbored a degree of denial about the diagnosis, she found herself feeling sad most of the time, often weeping, but only when she was alone; she did not want Aaron to know how upset she was by his diagnosis. She slept poorly, lying awake at night remembering fondly the many wonderful experiences they had shared over the years and thinking about the plans they had discussed for their future after Aaron retired. These included traveling and building their antique collection by going to antique shows around the region. They had both looked forward to having more time to pursue these interests, as well as to simply spend more time together. Now, all of that seemed uncertain, at best. Stephanie had little appetite, and lost about four pounds over the first month following the diagnosis. She had enjoyed being part of a book club, eagerly reading the assigned books and attending all of the monthly meetings, but she now found it hard to become interested in reading or to concentrate on it, and she missed two book club meetings in a row.

Stephanie and Aaron had always had an enjoyable sex life,

and she now found herself craving physical intimacy more than ever, even though Aaron did not seem as interested as in the past. When they did have sexual relations, she found it hard to be fully responsive despite her desire for closeness.

....

Stephanie's reaction to Aaron's illness reveals great anguish. In some ways, this stage of anguish can be difficult to distinguish from a depressive episode. Indeed, symptoms such as those experienced by Stephanie often lead to a diagnosis of depression. Many Alzheimer's care partners are given antidepressants to help them cope with these early reactions to the illness. At times, antidepressants can be very helpful, but at other times, they are not effective, often because the emotional reaction being experienced is not depression but instead is "simply" terrible sadness or grief. Differentiating sadness, or grief, from depression is critically important, although it is often difficult. This issue is discussed at length in the final chapter, "Understanding and Coping with Stress in the Family Care Partner."

Adaptation

The second stage of Alzheimer's grief is *adaptation*. This stage consists of the cognitive and behavioral alterations—the adaptations—that must be made by the family member in response to the changes occurring in the person with the disease. The relationship between the person with the disease and the family member is in a state of transition: the afflicted person has changed, and the family member must adapt to those changes and must herself change. The end point of this stage is the creation of a new relationship between the person with the disease and the family member. Before this is complete, there can be much instability, with important opportunities for personal growth on the part of the family member. But there are also significant risks for despair, the development of pathological grief, or other maladaptive responses (Bryant 2013; Schultz et al. 2006).

Struggling to Adapt to New Realities

Learning to cope with the changes in the person with the disease can be challenging at any point in the care partner's journey, but it can be especially difficult when the care partner is just beginning to learn to adapt to these changes.

....

Following a confrontation with her mother, who was upset and irrational, Cora stormed out of her mother's room. She went downstairs and jumped on an elliptical trainer. As she energetically pumped her arms and legs, she repeated to herself: "This is not my fault! This is not my fault!" She felt reassured by this but then realized "It's not her fault, either." She began to cry as she contemplated the many changes that had occurred in her mother since the onset of her illness.

....

Not infrequently, the effort to adapt to changes in the person with the illness can lead to significant tensions, as each member of the pair struggles with their new relationship. While it is important to encourage the person with Alzheimer's to exercise as much agency as possible, for as long as possible, it can be difficult to know how to determine a "correct" response to behaviors that occur during this transitional state. Adaptation thus involves a significant amount of trial and error.

....

A few times each week, Carla would visit her mother and prepare a meal for them to enjoy together. When they finished eating, Carla would frequently say, "Mom, why don't you go brush your teeth while I clean up?" This would cause Ruth to get angry and defensive. Carla did not understand why this was happening. She had taken education courses and read books on how to talk to someone with dementia and felt she had a grasp on the changing situation.

Eventually, and after seeking professional guidance, Carla realized that she was being somewhat infantilizing by asking her mother to brush her teeth. The fact that she did this lovingly did not change Ruth's response; parents with dementia can be especially sensitive to this type of remark when it comes from one of their children. It was suggested that Carla focus, instead, on having her mother help her with preparing the meal and cleaning up afterward, and on simply enjoying her time with her mother. She was advised to leave the hygiene issues to the private care partners who were assisting her mother on a daily basis.

Autonomy versus Safety

A central challenge for the family member at this stage is to determine how to help the person with Alzheimer's disease maintain her independence and sense of agency for as long as possible, while at the same time trying to provide support, assistance, and safety to someone who in many ways can no longer take care of herself. While this difficult dilemma often begins with the onset of the disease, it is at its most intense during this stage of adaptation; the person with the illness is now neither fully functional, nor completely dependent, either. As a result, the family member needs to adapt to the changing situation in previously untested ways.

....

Thelma had been diagnosed with Alzheimer's disease about two years ago. Her husband, Fred, had no cognitive impairments and was able to provide Thelma with all of the support and assistance she needed. However, when he suddenly died, Thelma's daughter, Wanda, quickly moved Thelma into her house. Fred's death happened in the early summer, and since Wanda worked as a teacher, she was able to be at home full time for almost two months to assist her mother with her loss, as well as the transition in her living arrangements.

However, when school reopened at the end of August, Wanda felt uneasy about leaving her mother home alone for most of the day, even though her mother indicated that she was perfectly content with that arrangement and strongly refused to have anyone come to the house for companionship during the time Wanda was at work. Thelma had a close friend who agreed to spend Thursdays with Thelma, but that left the other four days of the week when Thelma would be unsupervised for much of the day.

Wanda tried to persuade her mother to attend a day program for persons with dementia that was held in their town, but Thelma would not consider it. She insisted that she was fine staying home alone and had no use for such "simple-minded" activities, anyway.

Wanda felt frustrated and worried but did not feel that her mother's condition warranted forcing the issue. Thelma was still able to manage her activities of daily living, make a simple lunch for herself, and even do a few light household chores, such as dusting and unloading the dishwasher. However the dishwasher became a source of tension between them because Thelma had a great deal of trouble placing the clean dishes in their proper location. Wanda would become irritated with her when she could not find a needed dish or utensil, and Thelma would have no idea where she might have placed it. Finally, Wanda asked her not to put the dishes away any more, which seemed to hurt Thelma's feelings as she had felt she was being helpful. She continued to put them away for a while, probably not remembering Wanda's request. Wanda decided that she, herself, would simply empty the dishwasher before school in the morning.

One day, driving home from school, Wanda was shocked to find her mother walking down the road in a direction away from their house, about one-quarter of a mile from home. Thelma was very glad to see her, but was obviously quite upset. When Wanda asked about what she was doing, Thelma defensively said she had simply decided to go for a walk on a pleasant (but rather chilly) afternoon. With further questioning, Thelma admitted that she had been away from the house for nearly two hours, having gotten lost. She could not find her way back and was quite shaken by the experience.

Wanda again tried to persuade her mother to have someone come in to stay with her during the day, but Thelma remained adamant that she did not want that, and promised she would not go walking again; if she felt the need for fresh air, she would simply sit in the backyard. There were no more incidents for a few months. At a visit to Thelma's doctor, Wanda described the wandering episode and reported that she had since obtained a medical alert bracelet for her mother through the Alzheimer's Association, which had a phone number that could be called should Thelma become lost again. The doctor asked if Thelma, herself, would be able to call Wanda's cell phone if she needed her, or if she could call 911 in an emergency. Wanda was uncertain; her mother had never called her, and certainly had never called 911. After they came home from the appointment, Wanda showed her mother again where her cell phone number was posted and wrote it on a sticky note placed next to the telephone. She also wrote instructions to call 911 in an emergency. The next day, Wanda asked her mother to call her cell phone, to test her ability to actually do this. She picked up the television remote, which was on the coffee table with the phone, and began pushing numbers randomly on the remote. Wanda gave her the telephone and asked her to try again, but by this point, her mother was frustrated and was unable to carry this out. It was clear that Thelma no longer had the capacity to use the phone to make a call. As a result, Wanda came to the conclusion that she would no longer leave her mother home alone. She considered taking a family leave from school so that she could stay with her mother full time but realized that going to school each day was an important counterpoint to her evenings and weekends spent with her mother, and she did not want to lose that. Thelma would need to attend the day center or have someone in the home to supervise her while Wanda was at school. This caused a great deal of conflict between them, but since Wanda had become convinced that these measures were necessary, she was firm in her insistence. Reluctantly, Thelma agreed to a combination of going to the day center for two days a week and having someone come to the home two days, while her friend continued to spend Thursdays with her.

....

Wanda had tried hard to accommodate her mother's wishes and to support her autonomy, but it gradually became clear that this created a potentially dangerous situation, and finally safety took precedence over autonomy in her decision making. Throughout their time living together, there were many discussions—and, occasionally, arguments—about Thelma's growing need for supervision, as Wanda struggled to adapt to Thelma's declining abilities.

Dignity

At times, it is necessary for the family member to make adaptations in order to preserve the afflicted person's dignity.

....

One day Cora made spaghetti for Lila, her mother, who was in the moderate stage of Alzheimer's disease. Lila looked at the plate, took the spaghetti in both her hands, and shoved it into her mouth. Cora cried out, "Mom!," but Lila just shrugged her shoulders and kept eating. "I thought then that I couldn't take her out to eat anymore," Cora said, "I didn't want anyone to laugh at her."

....

As discussed earlier, one of the common symptoms of early Alzheimer's disease is disinhibition. This can create uncomfortable situations to which the family care partner must adapt:

....

Joanne took her previously mild-mannered and very polite mother, Eileen, to a restaurant for dinner one evening. As they approached their table, they passed an overweight woman with a full plate of food set in front of her. Eileen said loudly, "Is she going to eat all that?" The diner and her family sitting with her heard the remark and were obviously hurt. Assessing the harm to the overweight woman and her family, as well as how her mother would have felt about her inappropriate behavior, Joanne decided it was best to limit dining out. Joanne and her siblings still took their mother out to eat for a while longer but did so during slow, off-times in late afternoons.

....

At other times, the family member may make adaptations that can seem demeaning in terms of dignity but that provide comfort for the person with Alzheimer's.

....

One day near Christmas, Cora purchased a lifelike doll for her niece, Bethanny. Lila, Cora's mother, immediately became attached to it, thinking it was her real baby. She spent hours rocking and cuddling it and proudly showed it to others. Cora felt embarrassed for her. "In fact," she said, "when my husband first walked in and saw her rocking the baby doll, he turned red and said, 'Don't let her do that!'" Cora had been uncertain how to respond to the situation, but after deliberating about it, she came to feel that it was for the best. "I understood his feelings, but it appeared to soothe my mother and gave her something important."

Adapting to Significant Memory Loss: Learning to Live in the Present

One adaptation that every family member needs to make in caring for persons with Alzheimer's is the necessity of "living in the present." As the disease obliterates memory for past events, and the ability to think about the future is an abstraction beyond the abilities of most people with the disease, the focus on the present moment becomes a necessity.

The following article, reprinted in its entirety, beautifully illustrates the ability to live in the present with someone with Alzheimer's disease.

ZEN AND THE ART OF ALZHEIMER'S

I sat across the room from my father on Thanksgiving night. He looked at me pointedly. "What's your name?" he asked.

"I'm Mary," I answered.

"Mary . . ." he prompted.

"Mary McLaughlin," I said, wondering if he would recognize that my last name was the same as his.

"Mary McLaughlin," he repeated slowly. He listened to the syllables as they floated in the air. Then he shook his head. No, it didn't ring a bell.

My father, a few months shy of his 91st birthday, has advanced Alzheimer's disease. Though he still has good days, he has forgotten most of the things that just a few years ago he would have listed as evidence of a life well-lived—his three college degrees; his two successful careers; his five grown children; his 57-year-and-counting marriage to my mother. They—we—are all shadows now. Glimpses. Points of information that he finds fascinating and puzzling, but that evaporate almost as soon as they are spoken to him.

It's all lost.

I've played that Thanksgiving night conversation through in my head a hundred times since it happened and it stings every time I do. And then, with each replay, I continue through to the second part of our conversation until I get to the part that salves the sting.

"Well," he said warmly. "Welcome. I'm glad you're here."

"Thank you," I smiled back. "I'm glad to be here."

"I hope you'll come back," he said.

"I will," I promised.

I imagine that, had I left the room at that point and returned a moment later, we would have had the same conversation again, and I would have had to introduce myself once more to the man who raised me.

I'm headed to my parents' house for an extended visit at Christmas and I'm preparing myself for the reality that I will be a stranger to him every time I enter the room. My strategy is a simple one, lifted straight from 1971. Be here now.

I'm reminding myself that my father's past is gone to him and it's not helpful or comforting to him when I try to recreate it. "No, Dad. Remember this? See? Look. Remember?"

I'm also reminding myself that it's not helpful or comforting to me to look at my father and see only what has been lost. "No, Dad, remember this? No, Dad. No, Dad. No, Dad."

So, this Christmas will be a Christmas of "yes," as I engage with my father on his own terms, moment by moment, each one a new opportunity for discovery, engagement and connection. "Yes, it's nice to meet you. Yes, I'd love to have to seat. Yes, I think we may have been neighbors quite a long time ago. Yes, it certainly is cold outside. Yes, it's nice to meet you. Yes. Yes. Yes."

I expect to introduce myself repeatedly to my father this Christmas. I only hope that each time I do, he finds that he is pleased to meet me.

And if he isn't, we have another chance—another opportunity—another moment. Right here. Right now.

MARY MCLAUGHLIN (2013)

Adapting to Significant Memory Loss: Expecting the Unexpected

Significant memory loss can lead to striking and unexpected interactions with the loved one.

....

Mindy was visiting her mother, Blanche, who suffered from moderate stage Alzheimer's. The two were enjoying lunch on the patio of Blanche's house. Blanch observed that she had not called her friend Lorraine in quite some time. Mindy knew that

Lorraine had been dead for many years. She took a breath and responded lightly, "Mom, Lorraine died ten years ago." "Oh," said Blanche, "I guess that's why I haven't called her."

....

Adapting to the illness will eventually help the care partner absorb such remarks, and know how best to respond to them. Here is another example of an unusual response from someone with moderate dementia.

....

Mildred was a ninety-two-year-old woman with moderate dementia. One day, as her daughter Geraldine sat with her, Mildred began to wonder aloud where her husband was. Geraldine became anxious, because her father had died fourteen years earlier. Having read that the appropriate response when a person with dementia does not remember the death of a loved one is to redirect them into other memories or conversations, so as not to confuse or hurt them, Geraldine attempted this. But Mildred would not be redirected, and began to work herself into anger as she recalled that her husband always had seemed interested in Patsy, a neighbor whose husband died some years ago. Mildred came to believe that he was probably out of the house having an affair with Patsy. Geraldine's anxiety escalated, and she finally exclaimed, "No, Mom, Dad's not having an affair with Patsy. Dad died fourteen years ago!" Mildred was quiet for a moment before replying, "Well that doesn't bother me as much."

Seeking Professional Advice on How to Adapt to the Changing Situation

Sometimes, when adaptations are necessary, multiple family care partners may not agree on what the best adaptations might be. Trying to balance the changing needs of the person with Alzheimer's with the sometimes-different needs and opinions of different family members can be quite challenging. In this circumstance, a professional consultation can be extremely valuable.

....

Two daughters, Amanda and Diane, sought consultation to work through the decision concerning their mother's living situation. Their mother, Dorothy, lived alone in her house, two hours away from Amanda and several more hours from Diane. Amanda wanted to keep Dorothy in her home for as long as possible, which she felt could be accomplished by hiring a geriatric care manager and home health-care aids. With this type of support, Amanda felt that Dorothy could stay in her house for possibly two to three more years before running out of funds and needing to be placed in a facility. On the other hand, Diane wanted to move Dorothy into her home with her family, which included her husband and two pre-teen children, until Dorothy declined to the point that she could be placed in a facility without a full awareness of the move. Each sister had strong, and differing, opinions about what was best, but fortunately, they were able to put aside their disagreement and seek professional guidance regarding the pros and cons of each choice. While it was clear that both options were very reasonable (indeed Dorothy herself seemed quite satisfied with either one) the professional pointed out that, all things being equal, it might be better not to exhaust all of Dorothy's funds on in-home care, so that if and when the time for placement came, there would remain some private funds, which would permit a broader choice among care facilities. With this consideration in mind, Amanda and Diane agreed that Dorothy would stay in her own home for the next six months, with help, so that she could enjoy her garden, but when cold weather came, she would move in with Diane.

Recognizing and Appreciating Changes in the Care Partner as a Result of Adapting to Changes in the Person with Alzheimer's Disease

After struggling to make alterations to her own personality and habitual ways of reacting, in response to the changes that have occurred in the afflicted person, family members often come to an awareness that being a care partner has brought out new personal qualities, or qualities that they did not realize they possessed, prior to the illness. Often (but not always) these new qualities are positive, and they may carry over into other settings and relationships, as well.

....

Christine and Kevin had been married for nearly fifty years when Kevin was diagnosed with Alzheimer's disease. They had no children. Christine had always seen herself as a mild-mannered, even meek woman, content to permit Kevin to take the lead in most matters in their relationship. For example, Kevin would usually decide where they would go on vacation each summer; he would take the lead in decorating decisions in their home; and most nights, he would tell Christine what he wanted for supper, and if they did not have the ingredients at home, Christine would run the store to obtain them. Kevin would even select the type and color of the car to be purchased when Christine needed a new vehicle. But they appeared to have a close and stable marriage, with their mutual roles rather rigidly defined as described.

Unfortunately, Kevin developed significant apathy in the early stages of his disease, which only worsened as the disease progressed. He became quite content to sit in the house doing very little, when previously he had been someone who always kept himself very busy. His inactivity extended to not wanting to take a shower regularly, even though he had been fastidious in his personal hygiene before his illness.

These behavioral changes surprised, alarmed, and upset Christine even more than his memory difficulties. They also compelled Christine to take a more active role in managing their household, since Kevin no longer seemed able, or inclined, to do so, or to make any decisions whatsoever. Christine found herself coping with Kevin's passivity by becoming more active and assertive herself, but this was difficult and anxiety-provoking for her. Her newfound assertive decision making included deciding when

Kevin needed a shower, and coaxing, cajoling, or even demanding that he cooperate. She now made all the choices for their meals and tried to serve healthier foods than Kevin would have requested in the past. Despite the fact that she had never even picked out her own new car, she eventually found herself having to insist that Kevin stop driving, after he became seriously lost on several occasions going to places that should have been familiar. Although Kevin initially resisted her attempts to control him, she was unfailingly patient and kind whenever she was directive, so that their interactions were rarely unpleasant, and he almost always acquiesced to her guidance after some initial, halfhearted protests.

....

The changes in Kevin's personality caused by his disease led to an important adaptation on Christine's part: she learned to become less passive and more assertive. Although the unhappy circumstances of Kevin's illness demanded it, Christine found herself feeling pleased with the changes she had made and realized that her "new" self felt more empowered not only at home with Kevin, but also in other areas of her life, as well.

Acceptance

The final stage of grief is called *acceptance*. In this stage, the family member comes to terms with the changes in the person with the disease and gradually develops the ability to emotionally accept the new reality, with some degree of equanimity. Reaching this stage requires the family member to accept that the person who existed before Alzheimer's disease has been irreversibly transformed; it is this new, transformed person to whom the family member must now relate. Certainly, core elements of the original personality may remain, and it is vital (and comforting) to recognize those. But it is essential to acknowledge, at the same time, that the disease has transformed that person into someone quite different. For the family member, this means being willing and able to abandon his dreams and desires for the person with the illness to be anything other than what she now is. Reaching acceptance with equanimity also permits the family member to bid farewell, psychologically and emotionally, to the person who existed prior to being transformed by the disease. This is a critical outcome of this final stage of grief.

Occasionally, the transformation caused by Alzheimer's brings about new, desirable traits in the person with the disease.

....

Ellen's husband, Wayne, changed a great deal during the course of his disease. At first, Ellen would try to reason with him and correct his perceptions and interpretations. Doing this "made us both miserable." Finally, Ellen began to accept that she "was not married to the same man." She discovered aspects of this "second husband" that she could love and enjoy. Before his dementia, Wayne was a perfectionist, which made him critical of Ellen and other people. Because the disease stripped Wayne of his critical faculties, he began to praise Ellen for the simplest things, like the lunch she would make for him each day. Ellen recounted her providing care and this connection with the transformed Wayne as her "best hour."

....

Sometimes, however, the disease transforms individuals in ways that are less desirable. Acceptance of the transformations caused by the illness comes most easily when there has been a strong and positive relationship with the person before Alzheimer's disease.

....

Joanne felt that Eileen, her mother, would have been horrified at the angry and paranoid woman she became as dementia took over. Prior to her illness, Eileen was a much-respected citizen in her small town, where she had been honored by the local chapter of the Red Cross for giving more blood over the years than anyone else in its history. Eileen received dozens of letters each year in response to her own cards and messages to people on their birthdays, anniversaries, and holidays. Joanne said that in the more difficult moments she could feel more tolerant of Eileen because she had been such a wonderful mother and because, clearly, this was the disease, *not* her mother, as she saw it.

....

Joanne's very positive memories of her mother prior to the illness gave her the strength and compassion to be able to care for someone very different from the mother she knew. She knew that it was the disease that caused this transformation and felt that her mother—her *real* mother—had no hand in this tragedy. Joanne gained psychological and emotional fortitude from the knowledge that her mother and the person under her care were very different people.

Although Joanne interpreted the changes in her mother as wholly caused by the disease, other family members may interpret the emergence of new behaviors as hidden characteristics that the disease has caused to surface in this now-transformed individual.

....

Cathy was the care partner of Stella, her mother. Stella was an extremely intelligent woman who was also very self-disciplined and self-reliant. As the disease took over, Stella became very needy and required more and more of Cathy's time and attention. Cathy interpreted this trait as not brand new, but rather, as a latent characteristic in her highly self-controlled mother. Cathy believed that the disease had unleashed feelings of neediness and dependence that Stella had managed to suppress through rigorous self-discipline.

....

Although some people would view such changes as the result of the disease, Cathy believed that these changes revealed a suppressed aspect of her mother's personality. It is unnecessary to know whether, in fact, this neediness and dependence existed latently in Stella before being revealed by Alzheimer's disease; it is only important to know that Cathy interpreted it this way, and that doing so somehow helped her cope with the transformation in her mother, and, finally led to her acceptance of the situation.

Other care partners discern a "core self" in the patient, even in the end stage of the disease.

....

Although Lana's husband, James, suffered from advanced Alzheimer's and could no longer speak or understand speech, he still stroked her hair lovingly. To Lana, this signaled the survival of his sensual core self. "He knows he loves me," Lana said. "If you define him by what he used to be able to do, he's not the same person. If you define him by his heart, he's still here."

....

Here is another example of basic personality traits remaining even as the disease has significantly progressed:

....

Ellen described her husband, Wayne, as restrained, kind, stoic, and reserved. "He was always rather formal," she said, "even with us at home." As the disease progressed, he retained these traits. Even when he was unable to recognize Ellen and saw her as a strange woman in his house telling him what to do, he treated her with respect. At other times, when he recognized Ellen, he would complain that the "other woman" sometimes annoyed him, but he always treated the "other woman" with kindness.

Saying Goodbye and Other Forms of Closure

Nancy Reagan poignantly described the "long goodbye" her husband's Alzheimer's disease caused. Although the entire process of coping with the disease in a loved one can be seen as the "goodbye," it would seem that after gradually working through the stages of grief, and finally reaching a state of acceptance, with equanimity, a true "letting go" of the person with the disease can now take place.

Family members will sometimes choose to say farewell during

or immediately following a sudden "episode of lucidity" (Normann et al. 2002). Episodes of lucidity occur in nearly all persons with dementia in the moderate or later stage. Suddenly and unexpectedly, the afflicted person seems significantly more verbal, more connected, more insightful — in tantalizing ways, seemingly like the person earlier in life, or earlier in the illness. Why these episodes of lucidity occur is unknown, although their existence is certainly not in doubt. Many a family member has been greatly surprised and encouraged that the illness seems to have suddenly gone away and that the person who existed before the disease is "back." Sadly, the moment of lucidity passes after minutes, usually, and the person is again just as he was before the episode occurred.

Although the family care partner understandably hopes that the person with the disease will also experience the emotional significance of this moment — that this is truly an interpersonal and not simply a one-sided moment — it can be difficult to determine whether this is the case, for obvious reasons. Nevertheless, for the family care partner, these moments of "farewell" have deep emotional importance.

Being able to say "goodbye" to the person with the disease can be valuable, for several reasons. First, as the illness has progressed, it is clear that the person who existed prior to Alzheimer's is less and less present, transformed into someone who is profoundly changed, even if core features remain. The "goodbye" is therefore expressed to the person who existed *before* the onset of the disease. It is that person who seems to appear during the moment of lucidity, although that is an illusion. When the goodbye is said later in the disease, but not during a lucid moment, it is clear that the significance of the moment is for the care partner only, but that in no way diminishes its great significance.

The second reason that saying goodbye is important is that it provides the family member with a degree of closure and the opportunity to move forward psychologically with her own life. This is discussed further in chapter 6.

....

Lon's dad, Dan, was his hero. Growing up, Lon had idolized Dan, an energetic outdoorsman with many friends. Alzheimer's took that person away from Lon.

As the disease progressed, Dan became agitated and aggressive. He started physical fights with Lon, sometimes around the pool table. Father and son circled the table slowly, as Lon refused to fight his dad, and told him so. "Even though you know it's not personal, that he didn't really mean it, it still really hurts," Lon acknowledged. At the height of Dan's agitation, the family had to call an ambulance and have him admitted to the hospital. The doctors felt they could manage Dan with medications, but when the family arrived at the hospital, he had been physically restrained because his aggression could not be contained. For two weeks, no one could subdue him.

Gradually, with increasing medications and other interventions, the situation improved. The day Dan came home, he was disoriented and confused, flickering in and out of awareness, even in Lon's presence. They sat on the couch together. Lon talked with Dan, who stared off into space. But suddenly Dan "came to," and Lon felt he had his dad again at that moment.

Dan told Lon that he was unable to control himself or his feelings. He apologized to Lon. Lon told his dad "not to worry" about it and that he loved and missed him. Lon said, "I kind of said my goodbyes to him then. I did not think it would be, but that was the last conversation I ever had with my dad."

....

As noted, moments of lucidity often occur at unexpected times. Here is another example of a care partner saying her goodbye, during a brief lucid moment:

....

One cold winter morning Irene tended to her grandmother in the kitchen. Irene's mother and sister chatted at the stove while they cooked eggs, and Irene stood at the toaster. "I felt my grandmother staring at me and turned around," Irene said. "Her pale blue eyes were especially alert and intense, and seemed to express her awareness of everything happening to her. That intensity was unusual for her. "You feel for me, don't you?" she asked and stated at the same time. Irene nodded her head. "I can feel it," she replied. Irene recalled, "We smiled at each other, the toast popped up, and I turned around. My mother and sister had not heard us. When we all sat down at the table for breakfast, the fierce presence in my grandmother's eyes, from just a moment before, had faded away." Irene describes this breakfast as a bittersweet memory, a tender recognition of shared love, and yet, after that day, she felt an odd distance between herself and her grandmother. The moment was so profound that Irene was left with a sense of having said goodbye to her grandmother. At the same time, it imparted a strange ambiguity to carry such a significant memory of connection with someone who did not remember.

....

Although neither Lon's dad nor Irene's grandmother retained those experiences, for Lon and Irene, they were important last moments with their loved ones.

Even as the farewell is made, and the person who existed before Alzheimer's appears to have departed forever, that individual nevertheless lives on in the memories of family and friends. This can certainly be a comfort for those loved ones who remain.

....

Sarah described how, at the "celebration of life" for her mother, Penny, when friends and family expressed their memories of Penny, Sarah recognized how their feelings for her mother were still alive and present, and would always be so. She saw how much Penny had offered them when she was alive, and how, in this way, she too lived on in them. "Nothing is lost," Sarah said.

Chapter Six
Acceptance and Moving Forward

In the previous chapter, the three stages of grief—anguish, adaptation, and acceptance—were described. This chapter continues the discussion of acceptance and considers factors that help the care partner achieve that state, along with equanimity, a sense of resolution, and minimal bitterness. Reaching this level of acceptance will permit the care partner to move forward with her life.

As previously noted, acceptance is not achieved in an all-or-nothing fashion. From time to time throughout the Alzheimer's journey, there will be moments of acceptance; there may even be aspects of the situation that are generally accepted from early in the process of caring for a loved one with Alzheimer's. For some, true acceptance may not come until after the loved one dies; for others, acceptance may never come at all. Those family members who are unable to come to some degree of acceptance continue to suffer, not just from the loss of a loved one, but also from the sense of having been diminished or damaged by the process. This is a wound that does not heal with time, but one that remains with the family member indefinitely.

It is unnecessary to emphasize that acceptance does not mean that one feels positive, or even neutral about the disease. The Serenity Prayer, a fundamental tool of Alcoholics Anonymous, asks for strength "to accept with serenity the things that cannot be changed" (Sifton 2003). This is a good model for dealing with Alzheimer's disease, as well: Alzheimer's disease is certainly one of those "things that cannot be changed." Often, the distress that occurs before a family member is able to reach a level of acceptance is due to his continuing to hold out some small (usually unconscious) hope that the situation *can* be changed: that the disease will get better on its own, that the medication will work miracles, that a cure will be found soon, that the situation will improve if only the afflicted individual tries harder, or that perhaps it isn't really Alzheimer's disease at all, and so forth. In order to reach a level of acceptance with equanimity, it is extremely valuable for the care partner to become involved with the Alzheimer's community and to take advantage of all that this provides (see chapter 7).

There are a number of external factors or characteristics that promote the development of acceptance; the absence of these may make acceptance more difficult, but not impossible. First and foremost among the characteristics that promote acceptance is having a strong, mutual, loving relationship with the person who develops the illness. When there has been emotional closeness, and particularly when there is a pattern of open communication between the afflicted individual and the family care partner, the possibility of achieving acceptance is greatly enhanced. Going through the various emotions described here will be less complicated, and the end result will more likely be successful when there has been a solid, loving relationship, rather than a conflicted one. It is perhaps not surprising that those family members who have had difficult relationships with the person with Alzheimer's disease prior to the illness continue to have a difficult time during the illness, and often have the greatest trouble reaching a level of acceptance and moving forward.

Other considerations are important, as well. When the family member is less burdened by the concrete, day-to-day burdens of caring for someone with Alzheimer's disease, he is in a better position to process the emotional and psychological reactions discussed in this volume and more likely able to achieve a state of acceptance. Usually, anything that makes caring for the person with the illness less difficult will help the family member accept the situation more readily.

In addition, it is much easier for family members to achieve acceptance when the disease victim retains the ability to appreciate all that the family care partner does for her, and is able to express this with regularity. Unfortunately, as discussed earlier, many people with Alzheimer's disease lose this capability, often early in the disease. This makes the entire process more difficult and makes it harder (but not impossible, certainly) for the care partner to come to a level of acceptance of this sad situation.

Other factors that promote acceptance include having adequate assistance from other family, friends, or hired help, and having adequate time for one's own life and interests independent of the providing care role. Having sufficient financial resources to manage this very expensive illness will by no means guarantee emotional and psychological acceptance, but it can help to make a very difficult situation somewhat less trying.

Acceptance is more likely, as well, when care partners are able to find meaning and reward in the tasks (Quinn et al. 2012; Zarit 2012). Individuals who have an optimistic outlook on life in general and who have strong internal emotional resources manage any challenge more easily, including this one (Contador et al. 2012). In addition, having a heightened sense of self-efficacy has been shown to help family members find more positives in the act of providing care (Semiatin et al. 2012). Self-efficacy is having a belief in one's ability to accomplish difficult tasks and reach ambitious goals. It is an attitude, rather than a measure of accomplishment, although having a strong attitude of self-efficacy is usually associated with success in one's endeavors. An individual's level of self-efficacy may be a personality trait developed early in life, based on upbringing and life experiences, or it may be based on other factors, such as genetics. However, self-efficacy can be fostered through counseling or various self-help techniques, and it is a useful tool for anyone who is facing the difficult task of caring for someone with Alzheimer's.

As discussed in chapter 2, using psychological defenses is a universal human characteristic. Defenses were described as psychological "shock absorbers," which can help the individual face unpleasant or anxiety-provoking situations more gradually and more effectively. As family members achieve a degree of acceptance regarding their loved one's illness, they continue to use defense mechanisms, but there is often a shift to the so-called mature defenses, rather than the excessive use, for example, of denial or rationalization. Mature defenses can be viewed as valuable and positive personality traits that assist the individual in adapting to a challenging or unpleasant situation with equanimity. These more mature defenses will help the individual achieve a sense of acceptance of the illness. The mature defenses include humor, altruism, forgiveness, and gratitude.

....

Mel and Gloria were discussed in chapter 2, where defenses were considered. They were in their early seventies and had been married for more than thirty years when Mel was diagnosed with Alzheimer's disease. The diagnosis was given by a highly regarded neurologist who very curtly and unfeelingly told them that Mel was suffering from Alzheimer's disease, which would continually worsen over the next several years, at which point he would likely need to be placed in a nursing home. Mel and Gloria were understandably angered by the manner in which they were given this news, and they talked on the way home about the doctor's abrupt, unfeeling style, rather than the diagnosis he had given. This case was presented earlier as an example of the defense of "displacement": both Mel and Gloria "displaced" their emotions about the diagnosis onto the doctor's unfeeling style, so they didn't have to face, so abruptly, the devastating news they had been given.

Gradually, Mel and Gloria were able to talk more about the content of the message, rather than the manner in which it was delivered, although they remained angry about the doctor's attitude and refused to return to see him. Their displacement helped them to more gradually deal with the fact of Mel's diagnosis and prognosis. Mel and Gloria were able to rely on their close relationship over many years, and they talked very frankly with each other about the illness and its implications. Gloria vowed to Mel that she would do all she could to help Mel stay as well as possible, for as long as possible.

Unfortunately, as time went on, and despite Gloria's best efforts, Mel did worsen, to the point where he lost his ability to carry out any tasks independently. Gloria felt unable to leave him at home alone for any length of time. Although Mel needed a great deal of assistance with his daily tasks, whenever Gloria would provide this, he would verbalize his deep gratitude to her. He often expressed his concern that taking care of him was becoming too difficult for her, but she reassured him that it was not, and genuinely didn't seem to feel that it was. They had two daughters in the area who frequently came over and stayed with their father so that Gloria could continue in her bowling league, something she had done for many years and continued to enjoy greatly, both for the sport itself and the social outlet it provided.

One Sunday, at church, one of their friends pointed out that Mel was wearing one brown shoe and one black one. Gloria wanted Mel to do as much as he could for himself, including most of his dressing, and she had not noticed this lapse in her rush to get ready for the service. She simply commented, "Yes, he's got another pair exactly like that at home!"

As the disease progressed, Gloria and Mel made the decision together that he should go to an assisted living facility nearby, where his needs could be met by the staff, since the physical burdens for Gloria were becoming greater and her own health was failing. It was a wrenching decision for Gloria, but Mel seemed to accept the need for the placement with a degree of equanimity uncommon in this situation, once he was reassured that she would be able to visit him very frequently. He focused on this being better for Gloria, and therefore he felt very willing to do it.

Both of them emphasized to each other that he was not going to a nursing home, as the infamous neurologist had predicted more than five years earlier.

Gloria visited regularly, and both seemed to enjoy the visits, although Mel tired quickly. At times she would sit with him while he napped, but at other times, he told Gloria that he needed to rest and that she should perhaps go home. She would usually take his advice and leave, knowing that he offered this suggestion out of his concern for her, as well as his own sense of fatigue.

Gloria had been attending a support group for a number of years and derived a great deal of comfort from the other group members who expressed their understanding of the need for the placement. When one of the support group co-leaders left, and the group floundered for a time, Gloria volunteered to become a co-leader and to try to get the group going again on a more regular basis. She was quite successful at it, and the group co-leadership became an enormously important part of her life. It was clear that her altruism in this regard helped her as much as it helped the others; she felt very good about being able to assist newer group members with their difficult journey through the illness. She believed that she and Mel had "done it right," and she wanted to share that with others as much as possible.

After two years in assisted living, Mel's illness progressed to the point of his no longer being able to communicate intelligibly. He would smile broadly when she came to visit, but she could not be sure he knew who she was, exactly. Ultimately, Mel went on hospice care, while still at the assisted living facility, and eventually died of pneumonia.

....

Gloria had gradually come to accept Mel's illness, although it caused her enormous anguish, and she often cried when she was at home, alone. But their years of emotional closeness, his willingness to discuss his illness openly with her, and his ability to express gratitude were important factors leading to her reaching a state of acceptance about the illness, as well as her loss of Mel. Her ability to joke about it (her comment at church about his shoes was just one example of her wit), and her altruistic desire to help others going through the same struggle were indicators of her having reached this level of acceptance. All of this made it possible for her to move forward positively with her life in the face of her loss.

Not everyone is able to reach this level of acceptance, unfortunately. For some, instead of acceptance, there can be bitterness. Bitterness usually combines feelings of depression, anger, and feeling cheated. It can readily lead to despair over the situation. Despair is distinct from grief, which is a normal but painful reaction to having a loved one with Alzheimer's disease. Despair implies not only deep sadness, but also a sense of hopelessness that one will ever feel better. Other emotions that suggest that the journey has not been successfully completed include cynicism, remorse, and resentfulness. Often, the family member feels depleted by caring for their loved one with Alzheimer's, rather than having gained something from the experience, no matter how exhausting or sad it has been (Ott et al. 2007).

....

In chapter 3, the relationship of Marlene and her mother, Ethel, was discussed. After Ethel developed Alzheimer's, Marlene arranged for Ethel to move in with her and her husband, Joel. Marlene and Ethel had always had a somewhat contentious relationship; Ethel was often critical of Marlene and would frequently pick fights with her for no apparent reason. However, Ethel's seeming anger with her daughter became much worse as she became disinhibited as a result of her disease, and Ethel began yelling at Marlene, loudly and occasionally in public. Finally, Marlene moved Ethel into an assisted living facility, because of her increasing needs, in general, and her yelling, in particular.

The facility was almost an hour away by car, and although

it was not convenient (or pleasurable) for Marlene to visit frequently, her mother demanded that Marlene come on a regular basis. Marlene acquiesced, hoping that doing so would make her mother happy and cause her to be more loving with her. Although she rarely yelled at Marlene now, Ethel was often quite critical of the facility and frequently stated that she would never have put her own mother "away" like this. Marlene tried to explain to Ethel that she needed more care than she could provide for her at home, but this did not seem to register. Marlene usually left the assisted living facility feeling angry, depressed, guilty, and vowing not to visit as often, but before long, her guilt would start to gnaw at her, and she would take herself back again. Owing to her disease, Ethel was unable to judge how many days had elapsed between Marlene's visits, but whether the interval was short or long, Ethel always complained to Marlene that she hadn't seen her for "ages."

Marlene's husband, Joel, had hoped that Ethel's move to assisted living would mean that Marlene would soon resume her previously cheerful, attentive ways, but instead he found that the time she spent at the facility visiting Ethel, and her angry and depressed moods upon her return, were just as hard on their relationship as having Ethel live with them.

Marlene was also concerned and upset about the tension with Joel. Marlene hated the illness and felt she hated her mother for "dragging her into it." The situation continued, more or less unchanged, for about six months, when Ethel suddenly had a serious heart attack, and died several days later in the hospital. Marlene found herself struggling with a mixture of feelings, including relief, sadness, bitterness, and guilt.

Shortly after her mother died, Marlene was asked if there was anything she felt she had gained from the experience of caring for her mother during her illness. She paused for a long time, and then said, "No. Nothing. I'm just glad it's over."

....

Unfortunately, Marlene was not able to attain any degree of acceptance regarding her mother's illness, at least while Ethel was still living or in the immediate aftermath of her death. Instead of feeling pride that she had been able to ensure that her difficult mother was well cared for, or to feel that she had gained in any way from the experience, it was apparent that Marlene felt "used up" and resentful of the time and stress the situation caused her, and the impact it had on her relationship with Joel. She clearly saw the situation with her mother as all "give" on her part and all "take" on Ethel's, rather than the more positive, mutual concept of being a care *partner* to her mother. She remained stuck in a state of chronic anger, guilt, and depression, even after the concrete burdens of her relationship were ended by her mother's demise. Sadly, she seemed unable to move forward psychologically from that point.

Fortunately, it is sometimes possible for acceptance to develop in relationships that have been difficult over many years. Usually this involves significant personal growth on the part of the family member. In some situations, in fact, the disease may significantly change the dynamics of an entrenched relationship, and "soften" a previously fixed, dysfunctional pairing so that changes for the better can occur that might not have been possible without the disease.

....

In chapter 3, Tom and his daughter, Ginger, were introduced. After Tom's wife, Ann, died, Ginger became the primary family member involved with Tom's care. She was unmarried and lived nearby, while her brothers were both married with children and lived out of the area. Ginger briefly moved in with her father after Ann's death, to help him through the loss, then moved back to her own apartment, hoping that Tom could manage on his own after he adjusted to the death of his wife. However, it quickly became apparent that it was his Alzheimer's, and not his mourning for his wife that was making it impossible for him to function successfully or safely on his own. Ginger moved back with her father but continued to suffer a great deal of anxiety about the situation and feared that living with her father meant she would never meet anyone and get married, as her brothers had done. She returned to therapy, on the suggestion of her primary care doctor, and was able to talk about her fears and anxieties, and also her frustration over the fact that her father, although very much in need of her being there, wasn't able to show his appreciation and often compared her, unfavorably, to her brothers.

Ginger decided, with the help of her therapist, that if she had to live with her father at this point, she would make the most of it and would work on improving their relationship. She would try to help him realize that she was as capable as her brothers and deserved to have him treat her at least as well as he had always treated them.

This change didn't come about immediately, and Ginger battled her growing impatience and sense of annoyance with her father. However, as time went on, and his dementia worsened, he actually became more talkative than he had ever been, probably owing to some disinhibition that was developing, or possibly because he was getting increasingly comfortable with Ginger. He talked for the first time ever about his own poor relationship with his parents and his feeling that his older sisters (who were often left in charge of him as a child, since both parents worked) were overbearing and mean to him. Ginger found her anger at her father lessening, being replaced instead by a feeling of sadness for the young boy who had been treated cruelly by his sisters. She felt that this explained some of his favoritism for his own sons, and she gradually was able to feel a welcome degree of forgiveness. After this important interaction, even though Tom's needs were increasing, and Ginger had to do more and more for him, she felt less resentful—and more pleased with herself for being able to take on this challenging job. She also found herself learning (out of necessity) how to do certain minor repairs around the house. Although Tom had always done these, he was no longer capable of even changing a light bulb.

Ginger continued to care for Tom at home, with the help of hired care assistants during the day, and occasionally in the evening or on the weekends, when she wanted some time off. Fortunately, they were able to afford this, because of Tom's generous retirement savings. However, as Tom lost his ability to walk or even transfer himself from a wheelchair, Ginger no longer felt able to manage him at home, and reluctantly made the decision to place him in a nursing home. By this point, Tom was no longer able to determine where he was and didn't even seem to notice the change.

....

During the years of caring for her father, Ginger grew from someone who felt a great deal of conflict and resentment over having to look after him, to someone able to gradually reach a level of acceptance of his illness. She was able to move forward with her life in a number of important ways, making new friends, gaining a promotion at work, and beginning a relationship with a man that seems serious and hopeful. When Tom died, several months into the stay at the nursing home, Ginger felt much anguish but was also very pleased that she had been able to care for him at home throughout most of his illness. She had no regrets about any of her decisions. She felt she had gained from the experience, learning how to manage a variety of daytime care partners, learning how to do household tasks and repairs she had never handled before, and most important, learning how to forgive. She learned that, for her at least, forgiveness was critical in developing a new sense of maturity and freedom. She recognized that this was the most important accomplishment during the time she spent caring for Tom and felt that it would carry into other areas of her life, allowing her to move forward with a greater sense of her own maturity and self-worth, and a new ability to accept people more readily for who they are.

These examples should make it clear that there *is* life after Alzheimer's. If the family member has been able to reach a level of acceptance, then the life after Alzheimer's can proceed in a positive fashion, even though the family member is exhausted by the experience and remains deeply saddened by the loss. But, ideally, there has been the reward of personal growth, along with feelings of equanimity and resolution. The family member who has given so much to the task of caring deserves nothing less.

Chapter Seven

Connecting with the Alzheimer's Community

In order to achieve acceptance and to move forward with one's life, it is essential for the family care partner to reach out to the Alzheimer's community. This chapter discusses the multiple ways in which that is a vital part of the healing process for the Alzheimer's care partner.

One of the significant burdens of being an Alzheimer's family member, particularly as the disease progresses, is the sense of isolation that can develop. It is all too easy for the family member who cares for someone with the disease to find that there is little time left in the day to pursue one's own interests or engage in social activities with others. Even when family members are able to go out briefly during the day, leaving the loved one home alone, or in the care of someone else, they often use this time for errands and other solitary tasks. Family care partners often find themselves making quick trips to the supermarket, the post office, the shopping mall, and the like, accomplishing necessary tasks, and then racing back home to check on the person with Alzheimer's, or to relieve the helper who has been providing supervision during the time the family member has been out of the house.

As the disease progresses, it often becomes more difficult for families to go out with friends for a meal or entertainment. The person with dementia may no longer do well in a restaurant or enjoy or even be able to sit quietly though a movie. All too often, friends stop inviting the couple over for dinner, and even if they do extend an invitation, by the end of the evening it may become a very challenging experience, and a repeat invitation may be less likely to happen. It can also be difficult for the Alzheimer's family to have company for dinner, for many of the same reasons, and because of the extra work that will primarily fall on the already-burdened shoulders of the spouse or other family member who is the primary care partner. In addition, the person with the disease, owing to apathy, frequently has no interest in socializing or may actively resist it, because it is confusing, anxiety-provoking, and a disruption of the usual routine. Friends may stop visiting, or if they do come, stay only a very short time.

For many Alzheimer's families, all but the closest friends gradually tend to drop out of sight once the disease becomes manifest. Much of the time, this is because people don't know what to say or do around a person with Alzheimer's, feel uncomfortable, and therefore avoid the situation. Too often, this avoidance extends to the family as well, for a variety of reasons—discomfort; stigma associated with the disease, which often extends to the care partner; or simply a lack of awareness of how important it is for the family member to maintain these contacts, for example. As a result, family members frequently complain of feeling abandoned by their friends and associates, and bemoan the fact that they can go a very long time without having an extended interaction or conversation with someone other than the person with the disease, if that person is able to have a meaningful interaction with them at all.

It is an axiom of Alzheimer's education that the family member must ensure that she has adequate respite, contact with others, and opportunities to pursue her own life and interests outside of the role of care partner. Family members who spend some of their time *not* involved in care, who continue their relationships with their own friends and family, and are able to pursue their own independent interests generally manage the difficult task of being responsible for someone with Alzheimer's disease much more effectively. They are less likely to be depressed, are less stressed and exhausted, and have a more balanced perspective on life and the role that Alzheimer's plays in it. Although it is critical for family members to take the time for their own needs and interests, it is sometimes difficult for them to achieve this, for many practical reasons as well as for some of the emotional and psychological factors discussed in earlier chapters of this book. Nevertheless, trying to balance caring for someone with Alzheimer's disease on the one hand, and pursuing other areas of one's life, on the other, should be a goal for every family member.

As important as it is for family members to "make time for yourself," it is also vital for the family member to connect with the Alzheimer's community around them.

What is the "Alzheimer's community"? Wherever there are people with Alzheimer's disease, there is an Alzheimer's community. The community consists of those who have the disease, their family members and other care partners, and the professionals who are involved in their care. Nevertheless, this community often remains somewhat hidden, for a variety of reasons. This includes the stigma surrounding the disease, as well as the fact that until someone becomes associated with the illness (either by developing it or being a loved one of an Alzheimer's victim), one is likely to be unaware of the network, even though it exists all around. However, making a connection to this Alzheimer's community has great value to both the family member and the person with Alzheimer's disease. It is an essential step in moving forward from the anguish of grief toward a state of equanimity and acceptance.

The concept of disenfranchised grief was discussed in chapter 4. The grief of the Alzheimer's care partner is referred to as *disenfranchised* when he has been unable to have a full empathic exchange with someone who is, or has been, an Alzheimer's care partner. Nearly all care partners experience disenfranchised grief to some extent, and this can be a major barrier in moving forward with one's adjustment to the disease. This is one of the important reasons to connect with the Alzheimer's community; doing so will help "re-enfranchise" the sense of grief, when others who are, or have been, in the same situation can genuinely empathize with one's experiences. Through the process of emotionally sharing with others who have experienced the disease, an important transformation occurs in the family care partner that will ultimately help lead him out of a state of anguish over the loss, toward acceptance of the illness and the transformed loved one.

Although community support activities are vital for the well-being of both people with the disease and the family, not all of the resources discussed below are available in every community, particularly in more rural areas. However, they are not difficult to initiate. An experienced care partner, with the assistance of a local Alzheimer's professional or staff member from the Alzheimer's Association, will often be the impetus to create new community support programs where these have not previously existed. As the disease becomes more common, with the aging of the population, these community support activities are becoming more widespread, and they are needed more than ever. A detailed discussion of how to start programs of this kind is beyond the scope of this book; contacting the local office of the Alzheimer's Association is usually the best initial approach.

Alzheimer's Family Support Groups

One of the most common and valuable entry points into the Alzheimer's community is the Alzheimer's support group. The great importance of support groups is often not fully appreciated, and support groups are woefully underutilized.

Most support groups are for family members of people with the disease, and they generally do not include persons with Alzheimer's. The primary reason for this exclusion is that family members are reluctant to speak openly about their concerns and frustrations in front of people who have Alzheimer's. Since it is crucial that support group members feel as free as possible to express themselves, persons with Alzheimer's are generally discouraged from attending these meetings. In many areas, there are support groups for persons with early stage illness. These can be particularly valuable for the individual with early Alzheimer's disease (Yale 1995).

There are several reasons why family member support groups are so valuable. One has to do with the opportunity to learn about the disease, including its common symptoms and behaviors, and to gain information about how to understand and manage these symptoms from others who are coping with it on a regular basis. Support groups offer an abundance of helpful, practical tips and tools for dealing with Alzheimer's. For example, attendees can learn about what new symptoms to expect as their loved one's illness progresses, how to handle medical appointments, practical ways of assessing driving and dealing with driving cessation, recommendations about traveling, coping with the holidays, what to expect from medications, long-term care considerations, and information about local medication research trials, to name just a few topics that often are discussed in support groups. Commonly, the most helpful information offered in a support group comes not from the professionals who facilitate the group, but from those who are living with the disease on a daily basis.

....

Phoebe had been caring for her mother, June, for several years. June had suffered from Alzheimer's disease for about four years. For most of this time, her mother lived with her, after it became clear that she was not managing safely at home on her own, where she had lived alone following the death of her husband, five years earlier. June was now in the moderate stages of disease and needed considerable assistance with most of her daily tasks. Phoebe managed all of her instrumental activities of daily living, such as handling her finances and making sure she took her medications correctly. Phoebe had learned how to manage June's considerable "sundowning" (increased confusion and agitation that typically occurs late in the day) by giving her mother a snack at around three o'clock; putting on soft classical music, which her mother enjoyed; and occasionally taking her out in the car for rides when her sundowning did not lessen with these other interventions. Late in the day, June would often ask when her husband would be coming home, having no lasting memory of his death. She also would repetitively ask for Jack, Phoebe's older brother, who was married and lived in California. June often became quite anxious that Jack was late coming home from school, and no matter how many times Phoebe told her the realities of the situation, she could not keep this in mind.

June's sundowning had been going on consistently for many months, and gradually Phoebe became experienced at handling the typical behaviors that June displayed at these times. Gradually, her sundowning behaviors lessened, whether because of the progression of her illness, Phoebe's increasingly adept handling of the situation, or for other reasons.

During a recent support group meeting, Ursula, a new attendee, spoke about her frustration with her husband's afternoon agitation, irritability, and other behaviors. Ursula was aware that her husband's behaviors represented sundowning but was at a loss for how to cope with it. Phoebe described the situation with her own mother and offered a number of very practical suggestions to Ursula for managing the sundowning, based on her own experiences. She was also able to reassure Ursula that the behaviors would not last indefinitely, which was at least true in June's case. All of this was very helpful to Ursula, who became visibly calmer and more cheerful after listening to Phoebe's helpful suggestions. Being able to offer this help to Ursula was also very valuable for Phoebe; it helped her realize that she had, indeed, gained some important tools by being her mother's care partner, and that these were useful not only to herself, but to others as well. This helped her feel that she had grown in positive ways as a result of these experiences.

A second reason why going to a family member support group is so important lies in the interpersonal realm. Caring for a loved one with Alzheimer's disease is a unique experience: only someone who has cared for a loved one with the disease can completely understand what is involved on a daily basis. Conversations with close friends—as helpful as these certainly are—cannot replace the opportunity to interact with others who have had the experience of caring for someone with Alzheimer's, as well. Of course, it can be especially helpful to talk with a close friend who is also an Alzheimer's family member, but even that one-to-one conversation may not match the experience of being a part of an Alzheimer's support group, where there is the opportunity to talk with numerous people who have had or are currently having similar experiences. The group process itself brings thoughts, experiences, and feelings to the surface that tend not to come up in one-to-one conversations.

A phrase often used in connection with support groups is: "you are not alone." The importance of that simple concept cannot be overstated. Family members who care for a loved one with Alzheimer's often feel (before attending a support group) that their particular situation is so unique that no one else could possibly understand it, or help. This leads to feeling isolated and alone with the burdens of the disease. Even though a family member may be aware, intellectually, that others experience similar difficulties, the sense of comfort and reassurance that comes from interacting with others who have similar experiences is more powerful than any intellectual awareness can provide.

Even more valuable than learning that others have similar experiences is learning that others have similar feelings in reaction to caring for someone with the disease. The emotions discussed earlier in this book—anger, guilt, anxiety, shame, and, particularly, grief—are felt, to varying degrees and in various forms, by nearly every family member who cares for someone with Alzheimer's disease. Learning about this from support group members, as they talk about (and often display) their emotions gives the family member a sense of "permission" to have these same feelings herself. Realizing that others experience the same emotions, and hearing about how they cope with them may help the family member identify these feelings within herself for the first time. And for the family member who is already aware of these feelings (but perhaps uncomfortable with them), learning firsthand from others who are having similar emotions encourages a greater degree of comfort, acceptance, and further self-exploration than previously. This is a critical step in moving forward with the process of working through these difficult emotions.

....

Marian had been caring for her husband, Donald, for about four years. Donald has progressed into the late-moderate stages of the disease. He had previously been a voracious reader but was no longer able to comprehend reading material, so he had gradually given this up. He never had other hobbies, so he spends a great deal of his time now sitting in front of the television at home. He is unable to turn the TV on or off, or change the channel, so will watch—or seem to watch—whatever comes on the station that Marian set when she turns it on for him in the morning.

He is often irritable and seems somewhat depressed. He was given a trial of an antidepressant about a year earlier, but that did not seem to be helpful, and gradually, Marian stopped giving it to him, on the advice of his physician.

Donald's ability to use language in a coherent fashion is declining, and it is often difficult if not impossible for Marian to determine what he is saying to her. When she shows her bewilderment, or doesn't directly answer a question that he believes he has posed, he becomes quite short-tempered with her and will bang his cane on the floor repeatedly, in frustration.

Marian began attending an Alzheimer's support group several months ago. She tends to be a rather passive member of the group. She comes regularly, appears to listen attentively, but contributes to the conversation only infrequently. At a recent group meeting, another family member, Rose, spoke with great anguish about her husband's illness and how he has gone from being someone who loved hiking, gardening, and other outdoor activities to someone who does almost nothing, particularly since a recent fall and rib fracture has made it almost impossible for him to move around comfortably. Rose tearfully stated that she sometimes wished her husband would simply die, so that his meaningless life and misery—and hers—would be over.

Members of the group were quite sympathetic to Rose's feelings, and a number of other members acknowledged that they had harbored similar feelings about their loved one. Everyone in the group praised Rose for the devoted job she had been doing caring for her husband. Marian listened carefully to all of this, and then began to weep quietly to herself. When one of the group members passed her a tissue and asked if she wanted to talk about why she was crying, Marian stated, with much hesitation, that she had also experienced feelings of wanting Donald to die, but had felt terribly guilty and ashamed of those sentiments. It never occurred to her that others might feel the same way. She had never before expressed these sentiments to anyone, not even her best friend. As the group closed for the day, Marian lingered with several members, talking in the hallway afterward. In subsequent meetings, Marian began to open up much more than previously. She was able to acknowledge how bad she felt for Rose and her husband, but also, how relieved she was to learn that she, herself, was not the only one who occasionally wished her spouse would die, so the suffering would be over.

....

It is not clear if or when Marian would have been able to come to terms with her feelings about sometimes wanting Donald to die, if she had not attended the group, and learned that others felt similarly. This gave her a great feeling of relief, as it provided a sense of "permission" for her own difficult and (to her) shameful feelings.

In addition to providing a sense of "permission" for difficult emotions, learning that other family members have similar experiences and feelings helps reduce the sense of stigma surrounding the disease and its victims. The stigma associated with Alzheimer's was discussed in previous chapters. It was noted that the sense of stigma frequently extends, by association, to the family member as well. It has been shown that the greater the stigma felt by the family member, the greater the overall feeling of burden the family member experiences (Werner et al. 2012; Kahn et al. 2014). While attending a support group may do little to lessen the stigma felt by the general public about Alzheimer's disease and its victims, it certainly can help the family member feel more accepted and understood. It also helps the family member feel that she is not being looked down upon because of the illness, at least within the smaller circle of the group. She is able to feel more accepted and less stigmatized. Gradually, that sense of acceptance can extend into other areas of the family member's interpersonal realm, as well.

Occasionally, a family member might feel and express scorn or prejudice toward the individual with the disease, and verbalize these feelings in the support group. While these negative feelings are often associated with a dysfunctional relationship that may long precede the onset of Alzheimer's, the stigmatizing attitudes expressed by the family member toward her spouse or parent can be felt by the other group members as an attack on all of their loved ones. While the other group members may empathize with the sense of burden felt by this family member, the group as a whole is unlikely to support the scornful or prejudicial attitudes expressed. To the extent that the stigmatizing family member is able to hear and consider these different points of view, it may be helpful in modifying those views.

....

Audrey came regularly to meetings of the support group, but it seemed that her primary purpose was to complain about her husband, Will. She sounded worn out with the task of caring for him, both because of his dementia and also because of some chronic, stable medical problems that interfered with his ambulation. Listening to her talk about Will, it became clear that their relationship had not been ideal for many years but that their involvement in their careers and the lives of their children seemed to allow them to overlook, or at least avoid, the fact that there had been little warmth and a good deal of mutual resentment and passive aggressiveness between them for a very long time. As Will developed dementia, Audrey became more resentful and impatient. In the group, she would describe his symptoms of dementia such as his short-term memory difficulties, his apathy and lack of interest in activities, and his mildly disinhibited behaviors as if these were traits that were designed primarily to annoy her. She would claim that she never expressed any of her resentment to him, overtly, but it was clear that she was seething inside, and it was hard to imagine that this did not get conveyed in some fashion to Will.

As Audrey spoke, often at great length, about her situation at home, it was clear that members of the group were somewhat uncomfortable. The group facilitator tried to point out how frustrated and angry Audrey seemed to be feeling, but she was not able step back and look at these emotions with any psychological distance. It was as if her unstated response to this was, "Wouldn't you be?!" Several members of the group responded to Audrey's comments, although most were silent. Someone pointed out that Will couldn't "help it." Audrey immediately agreed that was the case but then stated that she didn't understand why, given his obvious impairments, he wasn't more cooperative with doing things as she suggested, rather than by trying to argue for his own point of view.

Listening to her descriptions of Will, it seemed as if she was describing someone with at least late-moderate Alzheimer's disease. When the facilitator had an occasion to actually meet Will and talk with him in another context, he was surprised to find someone who had only rather mild disease; he was not at all as impaired as Audrey's comments would lead one to believe.

After several group meetings in which Audrey recited her list of complaints about Will, it became clear that other group members were moving from being sympathetic to the struggles she was having to feeling somewhat more sympathetic toward Will. Although these sentiments were not expressed directly, the group did seem less responsive and sympathetic to Audrey's complaining. Although Audrey continued to attend the meetings regularly, she spoke less than previously, and the group seemed glad to shift the focus onto other topics. About three months later, Audrey spoke up at the group about her relationship with Will. She spontaneously acknowledged that she realized that she had complained about him too much, and had come to realize and accept that he was not able to help himself. She took up yoga as a way to try to achieve greater patience. The group was extremely supportive of her new stance, and one or two other members actually joined the yoga class that Audrey found so helpful.

....

It is impossible to say how much her experiences in the group led Audrey to shift her feelings about Will's illness, but it is clear that the group, while very kind to Audrey, had not been fully accepting of, or sympathetic to, her complaints. It seems likely that she was aware of their reactions and able to use this feedback—ever so gently expressed—to help her in modifying her own reactions.

Studies have shown that attendance at a family support group, often along with other support and education activities, can be tremendously beneficial to family members. Such participation decreases stress, is associated with lower levels of depression, and may even be associated with delayed placement in a nursing home (Mittelman et al. 1996). Much of the benefit of support groups, however, may be harder to quantify in a research study, but is quite evident from talking to those who attend regularly.

Family members will speak about the group as a "lifeline" at a very difficult time in their lives, as a vital outlet and connection in an otherwise very isolating situation, as the only place where the family member can feel genuinely understood, and as an absolute necessity in order to maintain sanity, just to mention a few of the comments that are heard.

Utilization of Support Groups

Despite their myriad benefits, support groups are underutilized, unfortunately. There are numerous reasons why this is so. One is that many family members feel they are not able to leave their loved one home for the length of time necessary to attend, and they don't have the opportunity or the desire to hire someone, or to ask a friend to sit with the person with Alzheimer's, so that they can attend the group. A few groups are able to provide supervision for those with Alzheimer's during the family support group meeting, but many are not able to offer this service.

Others who are reluctant to attend a support group indicate that they don't want to hear about the problems that they may face in the future from those who have loved ones who are further along in the disease course. This usually represents the defense mechanism of avoidance, which was discussed in chapter 2. Another reason proffered for not attending a support group is that the time or location is inconvenient. Often, however, these are excuses used by family members who have other, defensive reasons for not wanting to attend.

A final reason, and one of the most common, is that family care partners simply don't feel they *need* a support group. This attitude is particularly common among male care partners, but it is not an exclusively male phenomenon, to be sure. They feel that to attend a support group implies that they are having trouble coping on their own with the task of caring for a loved one with Alzheimer's disease. Some family members feel that they would not want others to think that they were having difficulty coping with the disease in their spouse or parent, or they may not even want others to know that the family member suffers from the illness. In addition, many people are simply reluctant to share their personal lives with strangers or may feel that to talk about the loved one with other individuals who are not family members is somehow disloyal. While these feelings are perhaps understandable, they are rooted in the stigma surrounding the disease and not its objective reality. Presumably, these family members would not feel reluctant to share that their loved one had a broken leg or suffered from heart disease.

Attending a support group regularly, as discussed above, is one of the best ways to lessen the sense of stigma that family members experience. Unfortunately, those who could most benefit from attending a support group are usually those who are least likely to attend. Addressing this basic paradox is one of the important challenges in caring for families with Alzheimer's disease, for there is probably no single activity the Alzheimer's family member can pursue that is more important than regularly attending a support group.

It is quite common that a family member who has expressed reluctance to attend a support group—not feeling it is "necessary" or having other rationalizations—will, once she has been encouraged to attend a few times, become a "believer" and a regular attendee. Skepticism about the benefits of a group is common, but it can be overcome once the individual realizes that the group is welcoming, friendly, provides valuable information, and is an important source of help and an invaluable connection to the Alzheimer's community.

Other Activities That Help the Family Member Connect to the Alzheimer's Community

In addition to regularly attending a support group, other activities can also be very helpful to the family member in building a connection with the Alzheimer's community. For example, getting together informally with family members of other persons with the disease can be very valuable and enjoyable. These informal gatherings can certainly help solidify one's sense of connection to the Alzheimer's community, particularly if they happen regularly. For this reason, group members are encouraged to have contact with each other outside of the support group.

Sometimes these get-togethers will include those who suffer from the disease; this is also a very important opportunity for connecting with the Alzheimer's community, and it is discussed below in more detail. But there is great benefit to be had in family members meeting alone, without their loved ones. This might involve just two family members who meet for coffee occasionally, or it may be a gathering of a larger group of family members who get together to enjoy a meal together, or pursue some other activity. In some of these gatherings, talking about Alzheimer's disease is prohibited, so that the family members can focus on those aspects of their lives that are not associated with caring for the disease. More often, however, that is not the case, and talking about the disease and how to handle it is a central topic during the gathering, just as in a support group.

Another activity that contributes to community building, in addition to providing other benefits, is attendance at educational programs for family members. Most chapters of the Alzheimer's Association, as well as many other health-care organizations, offer these programs throughout the community. Obviously, the primary goal of these educational sessions is to acquire additional knowledge about the disease, but the sense of shared purpose and the social aspects of these meetings may be equally valuable. It is interesting to note that, sometimes, educational presentations that are rated very highly by the attendees have content that is already well known to the audience. At these sessions, one can observe the frequent knowing nods and smiles of the attendees as the presenter describes experiences and feelings that family members commonly have. This process can have a powerful effect, by "normalizing" events and the associated emotions in the family member's life. This provides a sense of shared recognition and helps family members feel that they are understood and "not alone." These benefits are just as important as gaining new information about the disease.

Activities for the Person with the Disease and the Family to Pursue Together

The importance of activities with other Alzheimer's families, without the presence of the individual with the disease, has been emphasized, but there is also great value in certain activities that family members can pursue with the person who has the illness. Of course, almost *any* activity shared by a family member and her loved one with Alzheimer's is valuable, particularly if the activity is enjoyable for both. It is critical for family members and disease victims alike to realize that they can still enjoy doing things together, even in the face of the illness, and even if the activity is not likely to be recalled shortly afterward.

....

Sophie and Morgan lived together in a retirement community. Morgan had suffered from Alzheimer's disease for several years, and relied increasingly on Sophie for assistance of all kinds. Although he was very kind to her, he showed little awareness of all that Sophie was doing to assist him. He verbally acknowledged that he had Alzheimer's disease, although he did not seem to have a full awareness of the implications of that, despite his high intelligence and education.

Their community was located on the shore of a lovely, quiet pond, and the facility had a number of pedal boats available for community members to use. One day, Sophie packed a picnic lunch and she and Morgan went out on one of the boats. They had a very pleasurable hour or so quietly pedaling around the pond near the shoreline, letting the boat drift while they ate their lunch, and enjoying the fine weather before they pedaled back to shore.

They enjoyed themselves greatly, even though Morgan had difficulty with pedaling, as he didn't seem to understand how to do it.

Just one day later, at dinner with the Whites, another couple from the retirement community, Mr. White described how they had spent the afternoon out on the lake in one of the pedal boats. Morgan listened attentively to the story, then turned to his wife and asked, "Why don't we ever do anything like that?" Sophie was tempted to remind Morgan that they had done that very thing one day earlier but quickly realized that the comment would serve no purpose other than to embarrass him (if he then remembered) or start a disagreement (if he did not). Instead, Sophie simply said, "That's a great idea; we'll definitely do that."

....

Sophie described this brief interaction as an "epiphany" for her. She described being able to set aside the irritation and disappointment she felt over Morgan's forgetting their nice picnic on the lake the day before and was able to genuinely accept that the outing had been a success because of the pleasure it brought in the moment, even if by the next day, the memory of it was completely lost.

Activities that involve the family member and the person with Alzheimer's, along with other Alzheimer's couples or families, offer important additional benefits. Such activities offer an opportunity for persons with the disease to socialize with others who have similar circumstances and to feel that they "fit in" with a group of peers. Having people with Alzheimer's interact with each other and engage in pleasurable activities together can improve self-esteem and lessen the sense of isolation and stigma that individuals with the disease feel, even if they are unable to express it in those terms.

Family members benefit from such activities, as well. In addition to having another opportunity to interact with other Alzheimer's families, it can be quite valuable for family members to witness other families interact with their loved one with the disease. This can sometimes provide excellent modeling for those struggling with the task of interacting with someone with Alzheimer's disease. On the other hand, it can also be useful for family members to observe other pairs interact in ways that might be less than optimal; it is not uncommon for family members to more readily recognize inappropriate interactions in other care partners than to recognize similar behaviors in themselves. Seeing such behavior in another may help that family member modify her own behavior in a more positive manner.

Another benefit of activities that bring multiple Alzheimer's families together is the opportunity for the care partner to interact with persons with Alzheimer's other than their own loved one. Family members actually seem to enjoy this, and it is one of a variety of interactions that helps reinforce the connection to the Alzheimer's community.

The Memory Café

One of the most valuable settings where these interactions can occur is the Memory Café, or Alzheimer's Café. These are increasingly popular, recurring, local community gatherings designed to bring together people with Alzheimer's disease and their family members, for activities, discussion, entertainment, and the like (Jones 2010). However, as with support group attendance, those who might benefit the most from this connection with the Alzheimer's community may be the most hesitant to attend. This can be for a variety of reasons, including the stigma associated with the disease, the reluctance to be open about it with others, or denial of the disease or its impact. Nevertheless, those who are reluctant should be encouraged to at least give it a try, just as those reluctant to attend a family member support group need to be encouraged to do so the first few times. Many Alzheimer's families who didn't think that they wanted to attend Memory Café find that it has become an important part of their lives, once they attend a few sessions.

....

Katrina and Warren have been married for eleven years. Both had previous marriages that ended in divorce. Warren was diagnosed with dementia about three years ago. They each have several children in a neighboring state, who visit every few weeks.

Katrina and Warren have been attending the Memory Café nearly every month for several years. They drive nearly two hours each way to reach the program, occasionally staying over in a local hotel near the Café, in order to not have to leave so early in the morning, and to make a "weekend getaway" out of the trip. When asked why they are so committed to coming, Warren was quick to answer: "When I came into the room, it was like, okay, this is like home—big kisses and hugs."

As Alzheimer's disease progresses, the family's normal socialization patterns change significantly, with fewer social contacts overall, and only the closest friends staying connected. While this is not universal, it is common, and unfortunate, because both the person with the disease and the family member still need social contact—in some ways, perhaps, more than ever. This is one reason why it is so important for Alzheimer's families to develop a sense of connection with others who are in the same situation. But even for those who are fortunate enough to maintain their premorbid social patterns without much change, the value of connecting with other members of the Alzheimer's community is enormous, and it should become an important goal for every family member. The benefits of doing so will be great for the family member and the person with the disease, alike.

Chapter Eight

Understanding and Coping with Stress in the Family Care Partner

Caring for someone with Alzheimer's disease is always stressful. Even in the best of circumstances—such as a very close, loving, and mutual relationship; the absence of severe mood or behavioral symptoms; ample support and assistance from others; sufficient time and financial resources—family members nevertheless feel significant emotional strain or *care partner stress*, often called *caregiver stress* or *caregiver burden* (Adelman et al. 2014). Care partner stress can have a deleterious impact on the well-being of both the care partner and the person with the disease.

What Causes Care Partner Stress?

The most important cause of stress for all loving care partners is grief associated with the gradual loss of the person to the disease. Throughout this volume, the care partner's various responses to this sad reality have been discussed. Although a thorough understanding of this grief helps the care partner cope more effectively, no amount of understanding or psychological insight into the loss can take away the anguish of gradually losing a loved one to Alzheimer's disease.

The first part of this chapter examines the variety of factors that contribute to care partner stress. These include certain common features of the disease, as well as specific symptoms that are especially challenging. It also examines the relationship between the person with Alzheimer's and the family care partner, and the particular characteristics of the family care partner that may make him especially vulnerable.

Next, some typical ways in which family members experience the stress of providing care are presented. Some of the more severe consequences of care partner distress are then discussed, including care partner depression, mistreatment of the person with the disease, and care partner burnout.

The second portion of this chapter explores various techniques the family care partner can utilize to help manage the stress of caring for a loved one with Alzheimer's disease. Finally, the various types of professional help that are available to the care partner, should this be necessary, are discussed.

Common Features of Alzheimer's Disease That Contribute to Family Stress

There are a number of factors that are particularly stressful to many, if not most, family care partners.

Long Duration of the Illness

Typically, Alzheimer's disease lasts a decade or more, from the first appearance of symptoms (and the beginning of providing care) until death. This long duration, and the uncertainty of when it will be over, contributes significant stress to the family care partner. Most people can endure significant stressors that are of a known—and relatively short—duration, but the seeming "endlessness" of Alzheimer's is much more difficult to manage, psychologically.

Unawareness of the Impact of the Illness on Others

Most people with Alzheimer's have a diminished or absent ability to see or appreciate the many ways in which the disease affects the family member, as well as the many tasks that the family member must perform in order to keep the person with Alzheimer's safe and content. Often, the person with the disease may feel that there is almost *nothing* that the care partner needs to do for him, in spite of ample evidence to the contrary. This lack of awareness and lack of empathy can be very stressful for the family member who is working very hard to care for the person with the disease.

Concrete Burdens of the Disease: Financial Costs, Lack of Time, Physical Impairments

Alzheimer's is extraordinarily burdensome financially. Much of the cost of the disease is not reimbursed by health insurance. Even those expenses that are covered by insurance are rarely covered in full. That includes the costs of anti-dementia medications or other medications (for example, medications prescribed for neuropsychiatric symptoms), and doctor visits. Expenses that are typically not covered at all include the costs of hiring private care assistants; time lost from work by the care partner because of care demands; and the cost of long-term residential care, at least until the individual's own assets are depleted and Medicaid can be utilized. Spousal care partners, in particular, may witness a significant depletion of their life savings because of the many costs of the illness.

In addition to the financial costs of the disease, caring for a loved one with Alzheimer's disease extracts a huge burden in terms of time. Mace and Rabins have coined a phrase in their book title, *The Thirty-Six Hour Day* (2012), to describe the life of the care partner. There seems to be an insufficient amount of time to accomplish the many tasks the care partner must perform, in addition to the hours spent monitoring the person in order to ensure safety or engaging them in activities. Many care partners report that having no time left for their own needs after caring for their afflicted family member is one of the more stressful aspects of the role. This is particularly true for those adult children who have full-time jobs and their own young children, as well. These members of the so-called sandwich generation are especially stressed.

Finally, the disease can be quite burdensome physically. Inevitably, increasing physical assistance is required as the disease progresses, such as cooking a meal, cleaning the loved one's home, assisting with bathing and dressing, dealing with incontinence, and so forth. These physical tasks are easy for some care partners, but for spousal care partners who themselves may be elderly and perhaps not in robust health themselves, these jobs can be quite taxing. In addition, personal bodily care tasks, such as bathing, can be distressing for adult children, particularly those of the opposite sex.

Day-to-Day Variability

In Alzheimer's disease, variability from day-to-day, or even hour-to-hour, is a common but poorly understood feature of the disease. It may be that certain tasks that the individual can perform in the morning are impossible by late in the afternoon or evening, or (less commonly) vice versa. For completely unclear reasons, today, or this week, the person with the disease may seem especially cognitively impaired, agitated, or disturbed in other ways. Tomorrow, or next week, the situation may be much better, again inexplicably. This variability can be quite stressful, as the care partner never really knows what to expect or how to plan. Despite this short-term variability, however, the illness gradually worsens over time. Just as the family member is learning to adapt to a particular level of functioning and cognition, the illness will gradually worsen, and the care partner needs to adapt to a new, diminishing baseline.

Specific Symptoms of Alzheimer's That Can Cause Care Partner Stress

In addition to the features of the illness described above, there are a number of symptoms that occur in persons with Alzheimer's that can be particularly stressful for the family care partner. Many of these are mood and behavioral symptoms; family members consistently report that these neuropsychiatric features of the illness are some of the most challenging aspects of the disease with which they must cope.

Premorbid Personality and Behavioral Symptoms

What is the relationship of *premorbid* personality traits (that is, personality traits present before Alzheimer's) to the personality of the individual once the disease has developed? This is a complex subject, a full exploration of which would be beyond the scope of this book. However, it is often (but not always) the case that personality traits present in the individual prior to dementia will endure, in some form, once the person has dementia. An extremely polite, gracious individual will likely maintain those traits at least to some degree once he is ill. The person with a wonderful sense of humor is likely to retain that positive trait as well. It is sometimes said that the person becomes "more like herself" when she becomes ill, meaning that some of her long-standing character traits become even more noticeable in the face of the illness, and certain personality traits may even become exaggerated in the context of the disease. Unfortunately, however, this is often true with challenging or negative personality traits, as well. The woman who was always suspicious may become overtly paranoid. The man with anger issues will probably continue to be quick-tempered after the illness develops. Unfortunately, because of disinhibition, he may become even more prone to outbursts, or even physical aggression, over trivial matters. Certainly, these difficult character traits in the person with the disease can be a factor leading to significant stress in almost any family care partner.

Sometimes, however, individuals who have always been prone to anger, or perfectionism, or other difficult traits may become calmer, more accepting, and more mild-mannered in the face of the illness. While this is certainly welcome, it is not predictable (or common, unfortunately), and it is not a transformation that the care partner can bring about; it happens, or not, as a result of the disease.

Symptom Severity and Care Partner Stress

Just as the specific mood or behavioral symptoms that occur may not be predictable, their severity and responsiveness to treatment will also be quite variable. For example, many people with Alzheimer's will become mildly anxious secondary to the disease. While this is distressing, it may be only minimally stressful for the family care partner. However, if the anxiety is very marked, an individual may seek constant reassurance or may "shadow" the family member, staying closely at his side nearly continuously. This anxiety-driven behavior can become extremely taxing for the care partner. Likewise, mild suspiciousness in the context of the illness may not be seriously stressful for the family care partner, but if that suspiciousness leads to full-blown paranoia, with accusations about theft, infidelity, or the like, it is understandable that these symptoms can become extremely burdensome for the family member. Sometimes, psychiatric drugs—antidepressants, antianxiety agents, mood stabilizers, even antipsychotic medications—can be quite helpful in reducing difficult behaviors. However, psychiatric medications can have significant side effects, and it is often the case that the benefits of the medication are modest and can be outweighed by the adverse effects of the drug.

....

Dennis and Rowena had been married for more than forty years before Rowena developed Alzheimer's disease. Although they had experienced a significant amount of conflict in their relationship over the years, they genuinely seemed to feel a great deal of closeness to each other. Rowena had not been particularly prone to jealousy prior to her illness, but as she progressed into the moderate stages of illness, she began to accuse Dennis of having affairs with neighbors and with some of the women who worked in local stores. There was no objective evidence that this was true. Rowena began to accompany Dennis everywhere, in part because of her fear of being left alone, but also because she did not trust him to be around other women without her. No matter how cursory his interactions with women might be, Rowena would accuse him of being unnecessarily flirtatious and would see his generally polite behavior to others as an "obvious" sign that he was attempting to seduce them, or that he was already involved in a relationship with them. Rowena and Dennis spent many hours heatedly discussing this, and no matter how much Dennis tried to reassure her, Rowena would angrily accuse him of infidelity. She even accused him of having an affair with Susan, a neighbor who lived with her lesbian partner, Marie. When Dennis pointed out why this accusation was not only untrue but also quite irrational, Rowena concluded that he must actually be having an affair with *both* Susan and Marie.

After months of this behavior, Dennis brought Rowena in for an appointment and described her irrational accusations. At the doctor's office, she remained firm in her convictions about Dennis's infidelity. A variety of medications were tried over the next several months, but there was only minimal effect on this difficult symptom. Finally, exhausted, frustrated, and saddened, Dennis made plans to place Rowena in the memory care unit of a local assisted living facility. At first, she did not want to leave home, although she had a number of women friends who now lived in that facility. She believed that Dennis primarily wanted her to go there so that he could have more freedom for his sexual liaisons. Eventually, however, she agreed to enter the facility because she felt that she could no longer tolerate living with someone who (she believed) was constantly involved with other women. Dennis felt somewhat relieved to put this distance between them. The constant accusations about infidelity had become a source of extreme stress for him, and he was sleeping poorly, losing weight, and unable to concentrate. But he felt that, by having to place Rowena, the disease had defeated him, and he remained quite depressed and guilty for months after the placement.

Disinhibition

Individuals who are disinhibited have little or no "filter" governing what they say or do. Impulse control is significantly impaired in disinhibited people. Some types of disinhibited behavior are relatively common in Alzheimer's disease. For example, many people with Alzheimer's disease will make inappropriate comments from time to time. In chapter 3, the case of Roger was described. Roger made remarks about overweight people, including the new minister at his church, causing his family to eventually stop taking him there, and then to avoid taking him out in public, in general. Depending on the severity of this disinhibited behavior, and the family's attitudes toward propriety, this type of behavior can be a source of considerable stress on the family care partner, who may become embarrassed by the disinhibited remarks and then feel the need to maintain a constant vigilance whenever in public with the afflicted loved one.

Another form of behavioral dysregulation that can occur in people with Alzheimer's disease is *sexual disinhibition*: making unwanted sexual comments or attempts at sexual contact with others. Peter and his wife, Gwen, were discussed in chapter 3. As Peter's dementia progressed, he became sexually disinhibited with two different care partners whom Gwen had hired to be with Peter while she was at work. The impact of this on Gwen was further complicated by her unresolved feelings about her relationship with Peter prior to their marriage. But it is likely that this sort of behavior on Peter's part would have caused significant stress in almost any family care partner.

Other types of disinhibition can be extremely burdensome for family members, as well. In chapter 3, and again in chapter 7, Ethel and her daughter, Marlene, were presented. Ethel's frequent screaming at Marlene was an example of disinhibited behavior resulting from Alzheimer's disease. Ethel's screaming became very difficult for Marlene to endure and further worsened their already fraught relationship. This trying situation was an important contributor to Marlene's inability to successfully grieve over the loss of Ethel and move forward positively, as discussed in chapter 7.

Other Symptoms

Although behavioral symptoms are probably the most common causes of extreme care partner stress, cognitive and functional declines can also be very difficult for family members. As previously noted, many family care partners find it quite burdensome, both emotionally and physically, to have to bathe a loved one, particularly when there is resistance. Dealing with urinary and, especially, fecal incontinence is also a major stressor for nearly all care partners.

A very difficult milestone occurs when the person with the disease is no longer able to recognize the family member, either viewing him as a stranger or believing him to be a different relative; for example, the husband becomes confused with the father; a daughter becomes confused with the mother. This is, without a doubt, one of the saddest symptoms that occurs in this disease.

Relationship Issues and Family Burden

Care partner burden can develop even in close families with harmonious relationships. The enormous task of caring for someone with Alzheimer's disease almost inevitably leads to considerable stress. But when there have been difficulties in the marriage, or in the parent-child relationship, prior to the onset of the illness, the degree of burden experienced by the care partner is often significantly greater.

Discordance

The concept of discordance was introduced in chapter 1. Discordance is the uncomfortable but all-too-common situation in which the person with Alzheimer's and the family member disagree on the severity, or even the presence, of the illness. Typically, the family member is somewhat more realistic, while the disease victim tends to minimize her symptoms or be completely unaware of them. As noted, this often creates a considerable amount of tension between the family member and the person with the disease, and it is usually a source of considerable stress for the family member. When the degree of discordance is very great, the person with Alzheimer's may become very angry whenever the subject is raised, insisting that her family member is completely incorrect and that there is nothing wrong. This can have a very significant impact on care. For example, the person who is unable to see her illness clearly may insist on continuing to drive when this is deemed no longer wise; she may refuse to allow care partners into the house when her spouse or other family members are not able to be present, but feel that it is hazardous to leave her alone; she may refuse to visit the doctor for an evaluation or to take anti-dementia medications, and so forth. At times, the discordance is so marked and the person with the disease is so adamant about her wellness that the subject simply cannot be broached. This is hugely stressful for family care partners.

....

John and Isabel have been married for twenty-four years. Both had been married previously. John was an accountant, and until his cognitive symptoms began, he worked successfully for a large accounting firm. Unfortunately, as his memory and thinking began to deteriorate, he became less capable at his job, and finally, under pressure from his superiors, took early retirement.

John underwent an extensive evaluation for his cognitive problems. Initially, the assessment was not very revealing, perhaps because of his high baseline of functioning. Eventually, however, he was diagnosed with Alzheimer's disease. John was adamant that this was an incorrect diagnosis, and whenever his wife tried to discuss it with him, he would angrily insist that he had no such difficulties. He had always been prone to angry outbursts, and when discussing his supposed cognitive problems, he would become loud, red in the face, and extremely defensive. Isabel felt that she needed to drop the subject in order to maintain any degree of peace at home.

....

Isabel stated that the words *Alzheimer's* and *dementia* were never mentioned in their home, and that she and John had never had an in-depth discussion about his illness, even several years after the diagnosis. The complete inability to talk about his Alzheimer's and its effect on each of them has been extremely difficult for Isabel to endure.

Poor Premorbid Relationships

One might assume that individuals who have the closest relationships will suffer the most when one partner develops Alzheimer's. However, this is usually not the case. Of course, it is devastating when one member of a very close couple begins to show signs of the disease. However, some of the most significant stress occurs in relationships that are less than ideal in the first place. It may be that a family care partner who has an unsatisfying relationship with the person prior to the illness will be less able or willing to tolerate the burdens associated with the disease than someone who has an abundance of good feeling for the ill person. In some cases, family members who have been in very difficult or unsatisfying relationships abdicate the role of care partner to someone else entirely or else arrange for institutional placement sooner than might otherwise be necessary.

By the time a parent or spouse develops Alzheimer's disease, the quality of the connection between the afflicted individual and the family care partner has already become well established; it is, of course, impossible to rewrite the history of the relationship. However, it is sometimes possible, once someone has developed Alzheimer's disease, to finally address some of the unresolved issues between the two. It may be very important for a family care partner who has not had a good relationship with the afflicted person to attempt to resolve some of the problems that have existed over the years, and to do this before the disease has progressed to a point where it becomes impossible. There are times when the disease, itself, seems to make this reconciliation more possible, softening the previously frightening or unapproachable demeanor of the spouse or parent. While achieving a degree of rapprochement in the relationship certainly doesn't eliminate the stress of caring for the person, it can ease the burden considerably.

In chapter 3 and again in chapter 7, the relationship of Tom and his daughter, Ginger was discussed. After her mother's unexpected death, Ginger had become her father's primary care partner and moved in with him, despite their less than ideal relationship. Because of his dementia, Tom was unable to see or express any appreciation for all that Ginger was doing for him, and he continued to compare her, unfavorably, to her brothers, something he had done all of her life. However, as Tom's dementia progressed, he seemed to become more comfortable talking about his own difficult upbringing, which he had never discussed with Ginger before. Tom had two older sisters who were overbearing and frequently unkind to him, and who were clearly favored by Tom's parents. As a result of hearing about this, Ginger began to see her father's favoritism toward her brothers as a reaction to his own early life experiences. She was able to feel more empathy for him and was able to give up some of the anger and resentment she felt toward him. She was able to forgive him. It was Tom's dementia that seemed to allow his early life experiences to finally come to the surface, but it was Ginger's strong desire to improve the relationship with her father, before it was too late, that enabled her to establish a more positive bond with him.

At times, the reality of having to care for a loved one with Alzheimer's disease can motivate the family care partner to try to change the terms of the relationship.

....

Richard and Rita had been married for more than forty years, but theirs was not an ideal partnership. Rita was extremely critical of Richard in nearly every aspect of his being and behavior. Richard was quite passive, and it was clear that he felt fearful of and intimidated by his wife, who was strikingly similar in these respects to both his mother and older sister. His childhood had been difficult, and although he had hopes that marital life would be more rewarding, his choice of a partner who shared the demanding traits of his mother and sister led to him feeling chronically depressed and angry, although he never felt able to express this. Instead, he buried himself in his work, often covering extra shifts, and when not working, spending long hours in his basement on woodworking projects. Their two adult children long ago had given up trying to get Richard to be more assertive in the face of Rita's frequent criticisms. The children loved both of their parents but came to view Richard as a hopeless milquetoast.

When Rita developed Alzheimer's, the pattern continued. Richard did his best to care for her needs, but she frequently found fault with his efforts. Richard became increasingly angry and resentful of the manner in which he was treated and felt that he could no longer continue to put so much effort into caring for Rita in the face of her thanklessness and constant criticism. He finally decided that he had to confront her with this. Most likely, he found her less intimidating now that she had Alzheimer's, and this made it easier for him to approach her in this way. He told Rita that he had always hated being criticized by her, but that now, with all he was doing to care for her because of her disease, he found her criticism intolerable. He threatened to put her into a nursing home unless she was able to show more appreciation and to cease criticizing him. Richard did not really believe that her illness had reached a point where she needed nursing home care, but he threatened her with this out of anger. The threat was quite frightening to Rita, because her father had been institutionalized for dementia.

Rita was shocked at Richard's statements, since he had never before dared to confront her in this fashion, and this led to a long and difficult discussion about their relationship. Richard confessed that he had often thought about leaving her but never could muster the courage. He told her how he felt about his mother's and sister's criticism of him. She was quite aware of their treatment of him, having frequently witnessed it at family gatherings in the early years of their marriage. But she indicated that she thought this was how he expected or even wanted to be treated. This made him even angrier than before, and he yelled at Rita that it was the *last* thing he wanted. For the first time ever, Rita apologized to Richard for being so critical and promised to try to change. After this important interchange, Rita's criticism did not end, but it became less frequent, and whenever it happened, Richard was able to confront her about it, which lessened its impact on him. She would apologize and ask him to let her know whenever it happened again. On occasion, she was even complimentary, as, for example, when Richard would do the grocery shopping and prepare dinner. Richard was less angry with Rita than he had been since the earliest days of their relationship, and found himself even feeling pity for her because of her illness.

....

Although Rita's behavior didn't completely change after Richard confronted her, the fact that he was able to discuss it with her and have her express some regret and apologize was at least a partial reconciliation, after so many years. It made the situation easier for Richard to tolerate and also made it possible for him to continue to care for her and her growing needs. Had he waited until her illness progressed further, she may not have been able to understand or respond to him in the same way, and there would have been no reconciliation. It is important to note that it was their discussion of the issue, and her apology, that were so crucial to Richard, even more than the (partial) change in her behavior.

Family Care Partner Characteristics and Care Partner Burden

While there are some behaviors that would be extremely stressful for nearly all care partners, there are other behaviors or disease characteristics that might lead to significant stress reactions only in certain vulnerable care partners. What may be mildly stressful for one care partner might be extremely stressful for another; it is not always possible to determine why some react the way they do.

Different people have different abilities to cope with stress in general—whether that stress is related to pressures at work or school, handling a personal or financial setback, dealing with a personal illness, or caring for a loved one with Alzheimer's disease. Numerous factors account for the differences in an individual's general coping abilities. These include genetic or temperamental factors, personality, upbringing, and life experiences. Individuals with poor coping abilities may become easily overwhelmed by any stress; they may feel, before even attempting a task, that they will be unable to accomplish it or that they will perform it poorly. This lack of self-confidence causes the individual to assume that the tasks of caring for a loved one with Alzheimer's are beyond his abilities. He experiences extreme stress in the face of that (or any major) challenge.

Care partners who have a history of struggling with depression, personality disorders, or other significant psychological or psychiatric difficulties may have less effective coping abilities in general, and they are more likely to experience significant stress when faced with the challenge of providing care. For example, those with a history of depression are at greater risk to develop depression in response to the grief and other burdens of being a family care partner. This is discussed at length, below.

Some of the issues addressed earlier in this volume can also set the groundwork for experiencing extreme stress. For example, the family member who has been unable to move beyond some of the defensive reactions discussed in chapter 2 may be particularly vulnerable to undergoing extreme stress, because he continues to view the situation unrealistically and has not yet come to terms with the grief that is at the center of the family care partner's experience. Likewise, the family care partner who continues to struggle with one or more of the common emotions discussed in chapter 3—anxiety, guilt, anger, and shame—will likely find providing care to be extremely stressful, for similar reasons.

In chapter 3, the situation of Victor and Annabelle was discussed. Prior to his illness, Victor and Annabelle seemed content on the surface, but in reality, Victor was emotionally distant and often critical of Annabelle. When he developed Alzheimer's disease, he was unaccepting of the diagnosis, feeling that the doctor was incorrect.

Victor's getting lost while driving and abandoning his car on the side of the road while he wandered away in the rain led the local police to contact Annabelle requesting that she pick him up. They also took away his license. Eventually it became clear that Annabelle's fury at Victor over this incident reflected her long-standing, deep-seated anger at Victor for his treatment of her over the years. This created an enormously stressful situation for her as she contemplated her future with this increasingly impaired individual.

Unsupportive Family

While it is usually the case that other family members are a strong source of support and comfort for the primary family care partner, this is not always the case, unfortunately. Sometimes, other family members, residing nearby or out of town, can significantly increase the stress that the primary family care partner experiences. This can happen when other, less involved family members are critical of, or interfere with, the care that the primary family member is providing. This may be due to a genuine disagreement about how the situation should be managed. It may be that less involved family members have an incomplete or inaccurate sense of the severity of the illness or what is needed to provide adequate care. Sometimes, criticism comes from a family member who seems to feel guilty that he is not more involved; being critical of the job that is being done by the primary care partner sometimes seems to assuage some of the guilt over his lack of involvement. Lack of support or overt criticism can also reflect unresolved conflicts among family members that are being played out through the care of the person with Alzheimer's. This is particularly common when the primary care partner is a second wife or husband—a step-parent of the family member expressing disapproval—but it can also occur between siblings who have unresolved competitive or other issues.

The Impact of Stress on the Family Care Partner

Stress in Alzheimer's care partners has been shown to be associated with a significantly increased prevalence of depression and other psychiatric and psychological symptoms. Compared to non-care partners of a similar age, care partners suffer more frequent illnesses of their own, have a lowered immune response, make more frequent visits to the emergency room, and may even die at an earlier age than non-care partners (Richardson et al. 2013).

However, as noted above, there is enormous variability from person to person, so that what is stressful for one individual may not be stressful for someone else, or that which is extremely stressful for one person might be only minimally stressful for another. It must also be emphasized that the amount of stress experienced by a family care partner is not necessarily correlated with how loving or devoted he is. Significant amounts of stress can develop in the most, or least, devoted care partners.

Stress occurs in everyone, whether or not he is a care partner. What is crucial is how the individual copes with the stress he experiences. The desire to avoid stress is understandable, and it is appropriate for care partners to do what they can to lessen overly stressful situations, but it is impossible to avoid stress completely.

What does care partner stress "feel like"? That is difficult to describe, because it is different for everyone. For example, some experience stress as a low level of anxiety all of the time; others have a feeling of sadness, or less patience and tolerance for the everyday frustrations of life. People under stress tend to have less energy, and concentration may be impaired. The care partner may not be consciously aware, initially, that he is experiencing stress related to providing care, because it can appear quite insidiously as the victim's illness gradually becomes more manifest. But as the illness (and providing care) continues, the stressed care partner can become preoccupied with the source of stress—the person with Alzheimer's—to the point that it may become difficult for him to focus on other aspects of his own life. The family care partner often experiences a nagging, pervasive, unpleasant feeling: a sense that all is not well. A loss of a feeling of being in control—a feeling that events are controlling him rather than the other way around—is one of the stressed care partner's most common and uncomfortable sensations. Addressing the feeling of loss of control is discussed later in this chapter, when ways the care partner can help himself are considered.

It is a worrisome sign when stress begins to affect the care partner's daily life and has a negative effect on general functioning. One example is insomnia, caused by excessive worry about the afflicted person. Significant irritability, expressed toward the person with the disease, or toward others, or both, can also be a sign. Other stressed family care partners might turn to alcohol or other substances in an attempt to cope with the difficult feelings engendered by caring for someone with the disease. Not only do such substances actually interfere with the coping process; they will certainly have a significant negative impact on other aspects of one's life, as well. Other manifestations of extreme care partner stress, such as depression, mistreatment of the person with Alzheimer's by the care partner, and care partner burnout, are discussed below.

It can be helpful for the family care partner, himself, to recognize when the burdens of care have reached a level that requires a change in the care arrangements or when the burdens of care necessitate some outside professional assistance with coping. Care partners suffering from extreme stress will be unable to provide optimal care for the person with the disease. In addition, they will have great difficulty resolving their grief and moving forward toward acceptance. Such care partners can become "stuck" in a state of unresolved grief that continues to burden their lives long after providing care is over.

Depression

Are there any family care partners who do *not* feel depressed about having a loved one with Alzheimer's disease? The answer to this question depends on how depression is defined. As discussed in chapter 4, depression, in nonclinical terms, simply refers to feeling upset about something, and by that definition, it would be hard to find a family care partner who has not experienced depression about this terrible situation.

The confusion surrounding the term *depression* is understandable, but it is important to distinguish between the grief caused by having a loved one with Alzheimer's and true clinical depression, because grief, as has been emphasized throughout this book, needs to be understood and endured as an inevitable response to the many losses that are associated with having a loved one with the disease. Grief is not an illness; it is definitely not something to be hidden or disenfranchised, as discussed in chapter 4. It must be experienced and understood in depth, in order for the care partner to be able to reach a degree of acceptance and to then move forward productively with her life. On the other hand, depression (in the narrower, clinical sense) is an illness, an abnormal state of mind and body that usually requires some type of treatment to improve. While it is necessary to experience grief to be able to move toward acceptance and forward with life, depression, if untreated, interferes with (and, if severe, prevents) movement in a positive direction.

It can be difficult to determine if a care partner is suffering from depression or is instead in a deep state of grief as a result of the loved one's illness. Furthermore, grief is one of the more common precipitants of a depressive episode. Later in this chapter, some of the treatment approaches that can be taken with the depressed family care partner are reviewed.

Certainly, depression is one of the most frequent responses of the care partner to having a loved one with Alzheimer's disease. Some of those who are diagnosed as depressed may be suffering from severe grief, instead. Likewise, many of those who actually suffer from grief are given antidepressants, although these are generally not effective for the treatment of grief. Aside from the potential for adverse effects from medications, there is also the risk that giving a medication reinforces the belief that the symptoms are abnormal and need to be treated in order to lessen or be eliminated entirely. Because of the stigma surrounding depression and other mental disorders, this could lead the sufferer to feel ashamed of his reactions or to attempt to hide them from others. When grief is hidden, or "disenfranchised," it can impede the process of working through, and moving forward.

Distinguishing Grief from Depression

Although differentiating grief from depression can be difficult, even for experienced clinicians, there are some considerations that may be helpful in making this important distinction. In grief, the care partner rarely blames himself. He understands that the other person's illness is not his fault. In depression, however, there is often self-blame and a sense of being responsible for that which is not going well. While the depressed care partner may not feel he has caused the illness, he may feel to blame for some aspect of the situation. For example, he may feel that he is not doing enough to engage his wife in activities, thus hastening her decline. Care partners (indeed, people in general) who are depressed often have low self-esteem. While grieving care partners feel badly about the situation, depressed care partners, and depressed people in general, tend to feel bad about themselves.

Care partners who are depressed tend to have a more pervasive sense of gloom than do nondepressed, grieving care partners. Depressed individuals often suffer from a diminished or a complete loss of the ability to experience pleasure in general. Because of the social stigma attached to depression and its symptoms, the depressed care partner may not readily acknowledge to others or even to himself that nothing brings him any pleasure. He may not even fully realize this, thinking instead about activities he used to enjoy but has not pursued recently. By contrast, the grieving care partner certainly experiences great sadness in relationship to the ongoing losses of the loved one with Alzheimer's disease, but he is still able to experience some degree of pleasure in other activities. Indeed he may seem to crave those pleasurable activities more than ever, while the depressed care partner appears to have given up the hope of pleasure. Human beings seem to have an innate, instinctive need for pleasurable experiences, and unless someone is depressed, he retains that need for and ability to enjoy pleasurable activities, even in very dire circumstances. The loss of the ability to experience pleasure—a state that psychiatrists call *anhedonia*—is one of the most reliable indicators of depression (Dichter 2010).

Although it is fortunately uncommon among family care partners, the desire to end one's own life can come about when the care partner has lost the ability to experience pleasure and is unable to believe that he will ever feel better. Feeling a sense of responsibility for the person with the disease prevents most family care partners from acting on these feelings, thankfully, but when suicidal feelings are present, it is usually an indicator that the care partner is suffering from a serious state of depression and that urgent attention is required. Grieving but nondepressed care partners may have fleeting thoughts about dying, particularly as they contemplate the death of their ill loved one, but rarely have lasting suicidal wishes.

In order to qualify for a diagnosis of clinical, or major, depression, the suffering individual must meet specific clinical criteria (American Psychiatric Association 2013). At least five out of the following nine symptoms must be present, almost every day. In addition, one of the five symptoms must be one of the first two symptoms listed:

1 Depressed mood
2 Loss of the ability to experience pleasure
3 Fatigue or loss of energy
4 Feelings of worthlessness or guilt
5 Impaired concentration or indecisiveness
6 Restless motor agitation or the opposite, feeling slowed down
7 Recurring thoughts of death or suicide
8 Insomnia or excessive sleeping
9 Significant weight gain or loss

While it is certainly possible to have one or two of these symptoms as a reaction to stress, as mentioned above, the presence of five of them, nearly every day, is diagnostic of major depression. In addition, in depression, symptoms are often worse in the morning, improving as the day goes on. This "diurnal" pattern is an important signal of depression and cannot be accounted for by grief, alone.

Why Do Some Family Care Partners Become Depressed?

It is often not possible to determine why one care partner develops a depressive reaction, while someone else in a seemingly similar situation does not. However, there are a number of factors that may make depression more likely. A family care partner who has a history of becoming depressed in the face of other stresses, or for no discernable reason, may be more vulnerable, biologically, to this reaction, and is more likely to become depressed as a result of the stresses of providing care. Even if there have been no diagnosed prior episodes of depression, certain personality vulnerabilities might lead one to be more likely to become depressed in the face of the providing care situation. Indeed, the development of a depressive episode may be seen as one expression of extreme stress in a vulnerable individual.

Another factor, also mentioned earlier, is that family care partners who have had an ambivalent relationship with the person with Alzheimer's in the past may be more vulnerable to developing a depressive episode in response to providing care. Freud first elucidated the association between ambivalence toward the loved person and the development of depression in response to losing him in his classic essay, "Mourning and Melancholia" (Freud 1917). Harboring strongly conflicted feelings toward a family member interferes with the ability to properly experience mourning, and very frequently leads to depression (melancholia). This can be true if the loss occurs suddenly, through death, or gradually through Alzheimer's disease. In any case, developing depression in response to having a loved one with Alzheimer's is not a measure of the intensity of caring for the loved one; it has more to do with characteristics of the care partner.

Mistreatment

Other serious consequences can occur as a result of unrelenting care partner stress. One of these is mistreatment of the person with the disease by the care partner. This can take the form of physical neglect or abuse, or emotional neglect or abuse (Cooper 2006).

Physical Neglect or Abuse

Physical neglect can be said to occur when the person with Alzheimer's does not receive adequate attention to his needs. Examples of physical neglect include not providing adequate amounts of food or not ensuring that the afflicted person is able to consume it. Neglect of hygiene is a type of physical neglect that occurs when the person needs, but does not receive, assistance with bathing, or when the result of incontinence is not addressed promptly or adequately. Physical neglect can also be more subtle, such as not assisting a mobility-impaired individual to move from one floor or room of the house to another (when that is feasible, of course), or neglecting to take the person outside regularly, when that would be appropriate and welcome.

Ignoring complaints of discomfort or other somatic symptoms is another example of physical neglect. More serious would be ignoring significant pain or other signs of illness. Not providing assistance to get to the bathroom when requested, or not offering a drink of water when the person seems thirsty would also be examples of physical neglect. Another type of mistreatment is rushing or otherwise roughly handling the person while transferring or otherwise physically assisting her.

In situations such as these, the line between physical neglect and physical abuse is an indistinct one. Intent to cause harm certainly qualifies as physical abuse, but in some situations it may be difficult to determine if intent is present, or if there is merely physical neglect. Striking or kicking the person with the disease, twisting her limbs or grabbing her with a force that is painful are all clear examples of physical abuse. These acts are considered physically abusive even when they are done in response to the afflicted person's being aggressive herself, or when the care partner simply loses his temper and then is regretful and very apologetic immediately afterward, insisting that he did not "really" mean to hurt her. But physical abuse should also include carelessness and mishandling the person, even if there is no clear intent to cause harm. Whether acts of mistreatment are viewed as physical neglect or physical abuse may be open to interpretation, but the exact nomenclature is far less important than the immediate seriousness of the situation and the need to act quickly and decisively in order to protect the vulnerable person with Alzheimer's.

Emotional Neglect or Abuse

Perhaps more common, and more insidious, than physical neglect is emotional neglect. Emotional neglect occurs when the care partner pays insufficient attention to the afflicted person's emotional needs. For example, the person with Alzheimer's may indicate her desire for company and conversation, directly or indirectly, but the care partner chooses to pursue a different activity in another room, separate from the person with the disease. Of course, this does not mean that unless every emotional need of the person with Alzheimer's is met, every time a need is expressed, that the care partner is guilty of emotional neglect. It is clearly a matter of judgment and balance. One must take into account, however, that the person with the disease may have a limited ability to understand that the care partner is not able to devote all of his time and attention to her needs, and so it may be necessary for the care partner to explain to the person with the disease why he is unable to do this at this moment, if there is a possibility that this might be understood, on some level.

As with physical neglect and abuse, the border between emotional neglect and emotional abuse can be a very indistinct one. Sarcasm, for example, often expresses thinly veiled hostility. The care partner may feel that, since his conscious intent is to be humorous, the hostility behind the remark is acceptable, or even undetectable by the afflicted individual. Persons with Alzheimer's may have some difficulty understanding the meaning of a particular sarcastic comment but will have much less difficulty feeling the underlying hostility. Overtly critical remarks toward the person with Alzheimer's (for example, "You've made a terrible mess on the table with your eating; now I have to clean it up") are emotionally abusive, since the intent is to cause emotional distress. The care partner may feel that such remarks may help the person with the disease be more attentive to neatness while she eats, but even if that happens, for a short while (since it never lasts), the hurt caused by such an insult certainly does not justify the comment. While people with Alzheimer's may have a very poor memory for events that have occurred in the recent past, this does not mean that the care partner's insults are acceptable because they will soon be forgotten. Painful memories are often remembered longer than other events, and even if the content of the comments are forgotten, the feeling of having been criticized or insulted remains and further deteriorates the already very fragile self-esteem of the person with the disease.

Obviously, angrily yelling at the afflicted individual is emotionally abusive. Once again, judgment is needed, since it is a rare care partner, indeed, who has never lost his temper with the person with Alzheimer's, spoken more harshly than necessary, or said things that were hurtful and later deeply regretted. While one might wish that such events would never occur, it is almost inevitable, given the enormous stresses that most care partners feel. Clearly, however, if hurtful remarks are very frequent, the situation is abusive, and a change in providing care needs to take place.

Understanding the Reasons for Neglect and Abuse

Why do family care partners act at times in ways that are neglectful, or even abusive? Must one conclude that those family care partners do not care deeply for the person with the disease?

Are they sadistic, cruel psychopaths who enjoy inflicting pain on the defenseless? Are they seeking revenge for some real or imagined mistreatment by the person earlier in life? While sometimes it is necessary to draw such unsettling conclusions, most of the time the situation is quite different. The family care partner who becomes neglectful or abusive is usually a loving relative who is himself the victim of extreme stress and has lost control of his own impulses or his ability to make good judgments and behave appropriately in a very stressful situation. Most of the time, family care partners who have been neglectful or abusive are deeply ashamed and guilty about their behaviors. They need immediate help in managing the situation, and themselves.

Financial Exploitation and Abuse

At times, unscrupulous individuals who see an opportunity to enrich themselves at the expense of someone who is defenseless victimize people with Alzheimer's disease. Unfortunately, sometimes the perpetrator is a member of the family. Family members who feel burdened by caring for a loved one with Alzheimer's will sometimes take advantage of him financially, neglecting to return the change when given money to go to the grocery store, or writing checks to themselves from the disease victim's account when they are paying the monthly bills. Family members who do this justify such stealing by viewing it as "payment" for the services being offered, or feel that the person with the disease doesn't really need the money, anyway. At other times, persons with Alzheimer's disease are exploited by strangers who call on the telephone, offering to sell the person magazine subscriptions, insurance plans, financial services, and the like. It is an important responsibility of the family care partner to protect the afflicted person from such financial exploitation, and certainly not to be the perpetrator of such abuse, even when it involves relatively small amounts of money.

Care Partner Burnout

The end point of unrelenting care partner stress has been termed *care partner burnout* (Takai et al. 2009). Care partner burnout has occurred when the care partner can no longer cope with the demands and stresses of the situation, and there is an immediate need to rescue the person with Alzheimer's disease—and the care partner—from a situation that has become untenable and potentially dangerous. Care partner neglect may be a sign that burnout will follow shortly, or it may have already occurred. Significant abuse by the care partner almost always indicates that burnout has taken place.

When a care partner has "burned-out," he may declare that he is simply unable to continue, although because of the significant stigma associated with giving up the care partner role, he may be unwilling to acknowledge that he has reached this point, or may feel that he must go on no matter what, since no other options seem available. In fact, a burned-out care partner will often insist on continuing as a care partner, despite ample evidence that he is no longer able to perform the tasks adequately. Other family members or friends may recognize that something is seriously wrong more readily than the care partner does.

Signs of care partner burnout are often associated with significant care partner depression, and there will be the signs and symptoms of depression described above. Some burned-out care partners will, as noted above, become neglectful or even abusive. Sometimes the family care partner seems to lose the ability to feel concerned about the well-being of the person with the disease, even though she certainly cared deeply before. This is a serious sign that burnout has taken place, and others now need to step in, quickly, to assume the providing care role.

Other indications that burnout has occurred may actually appear in the person with Alzheimer's disease, herself. She may be more disheveled or unclean, may appear underfed, and is often in significant distress. She may seem frightened, angry, depressed, or anxious, or may simply crave attention. While these could be indicators of some other stressors, it is always wise to consider how the care partner is managing, when one is confronted with these symptoms in someone with the disease.

Can a care partner who has reached the stage of burnout return to providing care once relieved of the task for a period of time? If no changes occur, other than being freed of providing care for a number of days, weeks, or even months, it may be that the previously burned-out care partner should not return to the task. What happened before will likely happen once again, unless there are major changes in the caregiving situation. Typically, this means that much more assistance from other family members or paid care assistants will be necessary—not just temporarily but permanently. One of the dangers is that other family members may feel that all is well now that they have been taking a more active role, and that they are able to turn all control back to the original care partner. An equal or greater risk is that the burned-out care partner will feel, himself, that he is able to resume the task now that he has had a rest. Sometimes, when a care partner has reached the point of burnout, placement in a long-term care facility will need to take place. This is often because there are no other options for the person with the disease: for example, no other relatives are able or willing to assume the care role. If others had been available (and willing) in the first place, the situation might not have deteriorated to this point; one of the chief causes of burnout is not having any, or enough, help with the tasks of providing care.

Another, related, factor which can lead to burnout is the care partner who too rigidly feels that he must do the job completely on his own. Even if other family members are available and very willing to help, some care partners find it hard or impossible to accept assistance. Perhaps he feels it is his obligation (spousal care partners frequently feel this way) or perhaps he feels that no one else will do the job "properly" (that is, *his* way); and he is unwilling to give up any control over the task. The costs of this attitude can be enormous.

Coping with the Stress of Being a Care Partner

One of the goals of this volume is to help the family care partner better understand and manage the many burdens associated with providing care, by giving her a more thorough understanding of the psychological and emotional realities associated with the grief of gradually losing a loved one with Alzheimer's disease. In addition to developing this understanding, there are a number of principles that any care partner should seriously consider, in order to lessen the stresses and burdens of providing care. Some of these have been discussed already in the chapters above. While following these principles will certainly not make it easy to care for someone with Alzheimer's disease, they will help the family care partner work her way through this very challenging task.

---

1 The Family Care Partner Must Take Care of Herself *First*

Taking care of oneself must be the first job of any Alzheimer's care partner. This may seem either obvious, or selfish, but it is an important principle that is frequently overlooked by care partners. One can only be a helpful care partner if able to function effectively. Anyone who has flown on an airplane has heard the flight attendant say, during the initial safety instructions, that if there is a loss of cabin pressure, oxygen masks will fall from the ceiling; passengers are instructed to put on their own masks first and then assist any children with whom they are traveling to put on theirs. Why is this? In fact, if there were a loss of oxygen, the person who needs to help another must be sure that she won't pass out from lack of oxygen first. If that happens, the unconscious individual is of no use to someone who may need her assistance. The principle is the same with providing care. If the care partner does not ensure her own well-being, it will not be possible to be optimally helpful to the afflicted person who needs her assistance. It is not selfishness; it is sensible planning (Braff et al. 2002).

There are, of course, many components of self-care. To some extent, in fact, all of the principles that follow are ways of ensuring one's own well-being. However, in following the airplane analogy, maintaining one's own physical well-being should be considered at the top of any list. Alzheimer's care partners frequently neglect their own health needs while focusing on the needs of the person with the disease. Their explanation is often that there simply isn't enough time to do both, and while it is certainly easy to understand that point of view, it can be a dangerous one. It must be emphasized that a sick or deceased care partner cannot be helpful to the person in her charge. Care partners—particularly spousal care partners, who are likely to be elderly and therefore more vulnerable to physical illness—should visit their primary physician regularly for evaluation and monitoring. Blood pressure or blood sugar may become abnormally elevated due to the stress of the illness, or significant amounts of weight may be lost or gained. Other chronic illness may be worsened, either by the stress of providing care or simply because of the natural history of the illness, particularly if it is not attentively managed (Schultz et al. 2004).

Another area of physical well-being that the family care partner may need to address is difficulty with sleep (McCurry et al. 2007). Insomnia is a common problem for those who are caring for, and worrying about, a loved one with Alzheimer's disease. But chronic exhaustion from insufficient sleep makes any task, including this one, much more difficult and stressful.

What should the care partner who is having insomnia do to ensure adequate sleep? One thing the care partner should definitely *not* do is to use alcohol to try to improve sleep. While a drink of alcohol before bed may make it easier for some people to fall asleep, for many this is not the case, and increasing the amount of alcohol in an effort to get to sleep is definitely fraught with problems. Even if alcohol before bed shortens sleep "latency" (the time it takes to fall asleep) it is often associated with more frequent awakenings during the night as the level of alcohol in the bloodstream diminishes. Alcohol at bedtime will also lead to more awakenings for the bathroom at night, and getting back to sleep after awakening to urinate can be a difficult problem. In addition, regular alcohol intake can increase depression and of course lead to alcohol abuse or addiction.

It can be useful for the care partner having difficulty sleeping to attempt to determine the *reason* for the problem. What specifically about providing care is leading to anxiety? During the day, the care partner may be able to keep these concerns from her conscious mind by being busy or distracted. But at night, when trying to fall asleep, or return to sleep after awakening, these concerns or anxieties come to the surface. There may be specific worries or merely a feeling of being nervous or ill at ease. Some attribute this to not being able to fall asleep, but that is usually the result rather than the cause of the problem. Even though the whole experience of caring for a loved one with Alzheimer's disease is a cause of anxiety for most family care partners, it is important and helpful to try to determine those aspects of the situation that are most anxiety-provoking.

Earlier, the situation of Ginger and her father, Tom, whom we first met in chapter 3, was revisited. Ginger suffered from significant insomnia. As she thought about her father's growing cognitive impairment, she realized that she was going to be the one who would be primarily responsible for caring for him, because she was single, and that she would get little help from her siblings. This seemed overwhelming to her and caused her to worry, when trying to fall asleep, that she would end up living with her father forever. And she worried that she would never meet someone to marry. Because of her insomnia, her physician recommended that she return to a therapist whom she had seen in the past. In the course of several sessions, the therapist was able to help her identify and come to terms with her disturbing thoughts and feelings, and to find more positive ways of coping with her situation.

Finally, whatever psychological issues may contribute to sleep disturbance, sometimes the spousal care partner is kept awake at night by the loved one's restlessness, snoring, or talking during the night. If that is the case, it may be reasonable for the spousal care partner to consider sleeping in a different room from the person with the disease. It may be more important, overall, for the spouse to be rested, energetic, and fully attentive to her afflicted spouse, than to share the marital bed.

Similarly, physical exercise is an important tool not only for promoting good general health, but also for releasing some of the tensions caused by caring for a loved one with the disease (Loi et al. 2014). Many care partners report that exercising regularly is absolutely essential to their overall emotional well-being.

In chapter 5, it was mentioned that, at one point, Cora turned to exercise on her elliptical trainer to cope with the frustration she was feeling, and while doing so, came an important insight: she was able to realize that her mother's difficult behavior was not intentional, but due instead to her disease. This awareness, obvious in retrospect, was greatly relieving to her.

---

2 The Responsibilities of Caring for Someone with Alzheimer's Disease Need to Be Assumed by More Than One Person

Although there is usually one primary care partner (often a spouse or a daughter), the role of the primary care partner should be as the leader of a group of family and/or hired care assistants, and not a responsibility that she should assume single-handedly.

It is ideal for there be a team of individuals to regularly provide care for the person with Alzheimer's disease. This is a different view than many care partners, particularly spouses, have about the task. Those care partners often feel that they will only seek the assistance of another when it is, for some reason, impossible for them to manage the particular task. "I'll do everything except when I absolutely cannot" may be a very noble (and very common) attitude, but it is a recipe for extreme care partner stress.

In keeping with this principle, it is necessary for the primary care partner to learn how to recognize when there is a need to ask for a favor—and to become comfortable asking for it. This could be asking a neighbor to pick up something at the supermarket; asking a friend to sit with the afflicted individual for an hour or so while the care partner does an errand; or asking an adult child to accompany the care partner and the person with Alzheimer's to the doctor, for example. One of the most common hurdles Alzheimer's care partners face is their reluctance to ask others for help when they need it. But it is important to recognize that asking another person for a favor is generally a favor for both the person who asks and the person who does the favor: most people feel virtuous and happy when they are able to help others. The care partner will quickly learn if a neighbor or supposed friend resents being asked for the occasional favor, but most of the time, friends or family members are glad to be able to assist in this way; sometimes, it even "makes their day."

Another corollary of the principle of dividing the duties of care with others has to do with the vital importance of respite for every care partner. Respite means not only that the primary family care partner has time when she is not engaged in providing care tasks, but also, time when the primary family care partner can be relieved of the psychological burden of worrying about the person with the disease. Running out to the supermarket for an hour, leaving the afflicted individual home alone, and hurrying through shopping while worrying all the while about him at home, alone, is *not* respite. Of course most family care partners will be concerned about the welfare of their loved one even when they are not with him. But the family care partner needs to feel that, in the case of a more mildly afflicted individual, she will be perfectly safe home alone for the time the care partner is out of the house. In the case of longer periods away, or with more impaired individuals, it is necessary for the family care partner to have a solid feeling of trust in whoever is providing care during the absence.

Respite is different from "favors" in that respite, ideally, is planned ahead of time and occurs on a regular basis. Care partners benefit not only from having time when they are freed of the duties of providing care, but also from knowing ahead of time when such breaks will occur. Almost every worker appreciates knowing that, on the weekend, for example, she will not have to work. The same principle applies in caring for a loved one with Alzheimer's disease. Knowing that every Tuesday at 9:00 a.m., a hired care partner will arrive to spend the day with the loved one makes it much easier for the care partner to manage the other six days of the week. Too many primary care partners (at least in the earlier stages of the illness) feel that they can do the job singlehandedly, and they ask only for the occasional favor rather than arranging, from the beginning, for regular periods of care partner respite. Such care partners need to change their view of the situation from "is it *possible* for me to do this all alone?" to "is it *best* for me (and the person with Alzheimer's) to do this all alone?" An exhausted or irritated care partner is not in a good frame of mind to care for someone with Alzheimer's disease.

One of the most valuable forms of respite is an adult day program (Gústafsdóttir 2011). In an adult day program, skilled staff members attend to a number of people with Alzheimer's while the primary care partner goes to her job, or another activity, or simply has a period of respite. In a good adult day program, family care partners can feel that their loved one is safe. There is also an important benefit to the person with Alzheimer's: he has the opportunity to socialize with others, pursue activities that might not be possible at home, and have a level of stimulation that can be quite beneficial. Not all people with Alzheimer's disease enjoy going to adult day care, at least initially, but once the initial reluctance is overcome, it can become an activity that the individual anticipates with pleasure. In some situations, such as that of Ervin and Linda, discussed in chapter 3, the care partner will give up the program too soon, out of feelings of guilt, rather than trying to find ways to pursue it, knowing that eventually, most people who go to adult day care will come to at least accept it, if not actually enjoy it.

3 Family Care Partners Need to Maintain a Social Life and Interests Separate from the Person with Alzheimer's Disease

Many family members have reported that their ability to continue a part-time job, a weekly card game, volunteering at the local museum, or a weekly lunch with a group of friends has been extremely valuable in helping them cope with the challenges of taking care of a loved one with Alzheimer's disease. The care partner needs to maintain her own sense of identity, independent from that of being a care partner, and continue to pursue those activities that have been important to her. In most cases, this should also include social contact with persons other than the afflicted individual.

4 Family Care Partners Should Learn as Much as Possible about the Disease

Anyone who takes on the task of caring for someone with Alzheimer's should strive to learn everything she possibly can about the illness: the typical signs and symptoms, the usual course of the disease, common behavioral problems and how to manage these, the latest information about treatments, and many other topics. Knowledge is critical in managing any chronic illness, but this is especially true in the case of Alzheimer's.

Learning about the disease can come from many sources: for example, reading some of the many excellent books written for care partners, attending lectures or seminars at local hospitals or the Alzheimer's Association, or attending a support group. Increasingly, the Internet contains a wealth of material about Alzheimer's disease. Much of this is accurate and useful, but as with any online information, one should be certain that the source is reputable and up-to-date. The list of references at the end of this volume includes a number of useful and reliable websites, as well as a variety of books written primarily for care partners.

5 The Family Care Partner Should Engage in a Comfortable, Open Dialogue with the Afflicted Individual Regarding the Disease

Earlier, the significant discordance between John and Isabel regarding John's illness, and John's angry denial, was presented. This attitude made it impossible for them to have any discussion of the illness, and was tremendously stressful for Isabel. While it may sometimes seem that talking about Alzheimer's will create stress for the person with the disease, as well as the care partner, usually the opposite is the case. Family members — care partners and those with the disease alike — report they are much more comfortable once they have been able to talk openly about the illness. Of course, this must be done in a way that is not judgmental or further diminishes the disease victim's self-esteem. It may be difficult to "break the ice" on this topic, but once that is done, it is very beneficial for both parties to feel that the illness can be openly examined.

6 The Family Care Partner Should Talk about the Illness with Close Family and Friends

Some care partners feel that to talk about their loved one's disease with others is disloyal. While that sentiment is understandable, it is based on the false premise that Alzheimer's is something to be ashamed about, or hidden. Even though some significant stigma regarding the disease may occasionally be encountered, it is not helpful to let old-fashioned notions about the illness interfere with the care partner's sharing with important people in his life the facts about this very significant challenge he now faces. This is not to say that the care partner should openly discuss the illness with everyone he encounters; clearly it is a matter of judgment for the care partner to determine who should be told. But hiding something that is so central in one's life—being a care partner for a loved one with Alzheimer's—is both unnatural and unnecessarily stressful to the care partner, who needs the opportunity to receive support and understanding from those who care about him.

7 Family Care Partners Should Regularly Attend a Care Partner's Support Group

This was discussed at length in chapter 7, but it is important once again to emphasize the value of attending a support group. Many care partners are reluctant to attend a group, feeling that they do not need it, or that while it might help others, it would be of no worth to them. In some cases, care partners are open to going, but they can't leave their loved one home alone for the length of time it takes to attend the group and travel back and forth to it. This is a situation in which it may be necessary to ask for a favor from a friend, relative, or neighbor. Having someone spend time with the afflicted individual for a couple of hours while the care partner attends a support group is a wonderful gift, and one that the care partner should not hesitate to request, whenever necessary.

8 Family Care Partners Need to Find Activities They Can Enjoy Together with the Person with the Disease

A common challenge family care partners face is being able to identify activities that are appropriate, achievable, and enjoyable for the person with Alzheimer's. At times, the activities the afflicted person previously enjoyed are no longer possible. For example, a person who has previously taken pleasure in woodworking may no longer be able to use power tools safely; another person may have enjoyed doing crossword puzzles but now may no longer have the necessary vocabulary or problem-solving skills. It is important not to try to have the person attempt tasks that are no longer within her capabilities; this only becomes another frustration or failure experience for someone who has already experienced many other frustrations and failures.

Care partners should take careful note of those abilities that have been preserved in the person with the disease and focus on activities that make use of capacities that remain. Examples include listening to music, or enjoying paintings or other artworks in a museum. The ability to appreciate music and art (for someone who has previously enjoyed these activities) appears to involve parts of the brain that do not deteriorate until later in the disease, compared with short-term memory or the ability to perform complex tasks. Other activities that do not rely on short-term memory, and particularly those that may tap into long-term memory stores or long-standing areas of interest can be particularly enjoyable for someone with Alzheimer's disease. Examples include watching a sporting event, live or on television; sitting on the beach; going for drives in the country; having a snack of some comfort food; looking at old family photo albums; watching old movies on television; visiting with pets or very young children; and simple gardening. Finding these activities and pursuing them relies on the motivation and creativity of the primary family care partner. The person with the disease is usually no longer able to initiate this type of spontaneous activity.

However, in addition to the importance of identifying suitable activities for the person with the disease, it is critical to find activities that the afflicted individual and the family care partner can enjoy *together*. This can be one of the most positive ways to lessen stress in the providing care situation. Of course, these mutually enjoyable activities will be different for every pair. One pursuit, however, that is particularly valuable in this regard is walking together. Not only is there pleasure in the activity itself, but also, walking together promotes another crucially important activity: talking. Many couples find that a daily stroll is not only an enjoyable opportunity to experience the outdoors and get some valuable exercise; it is also an opportunity to casually converse together. It is hard to know if there is more benefit from the walking or the talking, but when combined, this is a wonderful activity for both the person with the disease, and his family care partner.

9 Family Care Partners Need to Find and Celebrate the Positive Aspects of Providing Care

While having a loved one with Alzheimer's and being a family care partner is not a task that anyone would choose, and while there are many very difficult aspects to the undertaking, it is not all negative. Nearly every care partner, except perhaps those who are in highly conflicted relationships with the afflicted person or are already severely stressed, depressed, or burned out, can point to positive aspects of the undertaking. When asked to cite what has been positive about being a care partner (a very useful exercise that care partners should practice on themselves), some will indicate that their love for their family member has grown as a result; others will say that they have learned, for the first time, the art of patience; others will talk about the many tasks they have been forced to master that they had never attempted previously—and did not realize they possessed the capability to undertake (for example, managing the finances, learning to cook, becoming proficient at household repairs, and so forth). Some will focus on how much they have enjoyed some of the activities they do regularly with the afflicted person—going for a walk, listening to music together, car rides. Others indicate that being a care partner has brought them closer to their religion, and they have learned how much comfort that can bring. Still others will simply indicate that they have learned that they can survive and prosper in spite of being saddled with such an enormous task.

Research has shown (and common sense reinforces) that being able to find and focus on the positives of providing care helps the family member endure the task with greater equanimity, less stress, and less depression (Cohen et al. 2002). Of course, this is generally true with any difficult activity: being able to see the benefits it offers makes it much easier to undertake. One does not need to minimize or ignore the difficult aspects of caring for a loved one with the disease or deny the enormous sense of grief that is an inevitable accompaniment of this experience. It is a matter of balance.

10 Family Care Partners Need to Experience a Sense of Control

People who have a very strong need to feel "in control" tend to have a very difficult time as Alzheimer's care partners. The nature of Alzheimer's is that the *disease* is generally in control and certainly not the care partner. For example, the family care partner may hope that the person with the illness is going to have a "good day" today, because company is coming over or because there is a doctor's appointment, but the day may end up being a very difficult one, perhaps because the afflicted individual has seemed more confused, more depressed, more irritable, more contrary, or more distracted, for unclear reasons. As another example, the family care partner may wish to spend some time with the person with the illness sorting through her belongings, in order to clean up and discard unwanted or unneeded items. On a good day, she may be very cooperative and helpful with this activity, but on the day in question, again for unpredictable reasons, the person with the disease may easily become preoccupied with other matters, won't consider giving up any items, or simply cannot attend to the task at all. Although the care partner may have had one plan in mind, the disease forced an unexpected change in the day's agenda. In both examples, the behavior of the person with the disease was unpredictable—that is a central feature of Alzheimer's. When behaviors and the general events of the day are so difficult to know ahead of time, it is easy to see why care partners can experience an uncomfortable sense of not being in control.

One of the most important tasks for the family care partner—particularly those who have a high need for control—is to determine which aspects of the situation she is able to predict or control, and to focus on those, while recognizing and accepting the many aspects of the care situation that are *not* in her control. Too often, care partners become angry, feeling that the person with the disease is purposely thwarting their need for control, but this is, of course, not the case.

Although it is the disease, and not the family member who is in control, the care partner may have some limited influence over the situation. For example, the day before an important event is planned, she can try to see that the person with the disease gets adequate sleep at night; this will help the afflicted individual function better than he would have functioned after a poor night's sleep. Although the family care partner cannot insure that the person with the disease will fall asleep and remain asleep on a given night, she can try to set the conditions for this to be most likely to happen, by engaging the individual in physical activity during the day, and helping him to wind down in the evening after dinner by playing soft music, or avoiding distracting television programs or the like. All of this may work, or not—the disease will have the "final say."

The only aspect of providing care that the family member can truly control is her *own* behavior and emotional reactions. For example, she can determine when she will and will not be the one who is providing care, by arranging regular periods of respite when other helpers, family or hired, are entirely responsible. It is extremely important for the family care partner to have regular, predictable periods when she is not responsible for providing care. One of the many benefits of scheduled respite is that during these times, the care partner can regain her sense of control over her own life, at least during these periods themselves.

The other aspect of the situation that the family member can control—at least to some degree—is her emotional reactions to the situation. She must understand and become comfortable with the loss of control that the disease causes and recognize and accept those many aspects of the situation over which she has very limited or no influence. It may be very difficult for the care partner who needs to be in control to achieve this state of mind, but it is certainly a worthwhile effort.

11 Family Care Partners Should Employ Relaxation Techniques to Help Lessen the Stresses of Providing Care

There are a variety of useful relaxation techniques that individuals can employ to try to reduce the stress and tension of being a care partner. Even those who have never felt that such self-help techniques would be useful or necessary should at least become familiar with some of the principles of relaxation training, keeping in mind that a relaxed care partner is a better care partner. There are a variety of relaxation techniques available, including progressive muscle relaxation, visualization, meditation, massage, and yoga. One especially useful technique that has become popular in recent years is called *mindfulness*.

Mindfulness teaches the individual to bring full attention to the moment at hand. Thoughts and feelings are observed as if from a distance, without making any judgments on them, positive or negative. It is a method of "living in the present." Busy thoughts, daydreams, emotions, to-do lists, memories of the past, and anxieties about the future all interfere with having a tranquil mind and body at ease in the present moment. Mindfulness can be viewed as a Westernized version of Eastern meditation traditions; as adapted for use in this culture, it is a type of positive psychology. Research has shown that the practice of mindfulness reduces stress and promotes inner peace and positive emotions, and it has been demonstrated to be a useful coping technique for dealing with the challenges of being an Alzheimer's care partner (Oken et al. 2010; Whitebird et al. 2013).

One of the important characteristics of mindfulness is its focus on the present. In caring for someone with Alzheimer's disease, this is particularly valuable because, beyond the earliest stages of the disease, the afflicted person lives in the present as well: the past is no longer recalled, and the future is too abstract a concept to consider. Therefore, mindfulness can help facilitate the care partner's ability to relate to his loved one in the present moment. Being present in a positive and tranquil way for another person is a powerful tool.

In chapter 5, the case of Sarah and her mother was presented. Sarah's decision to be joyful when visiting her mother created happiness in her mother. "Every time I visited my mother, she would break out into a big smile. It's a powerful gift to give to someone, to always be happy to see them and spend time with them."

12 The Family Care Partner Needs to Know When She Has Reached Her Limits, and Act Accordingly

There frequently will come a point, usually after years of caregiving, when the care partner feels no longer able to continue the task. It may be that she has "burned out"; or it may be that the physical and emotional demands of the task have simply become too great for her to be able to continue. Too often, care partners will push themselves beyond this point, feeling either that there are no practical options or that it would be shameful or disloyal for them to "give up." This attitude, while understandable, leads to enormous distress for the care partner and can lead to a potentially dangerous situation for the person with the disease. Care partners need to understand that it is neither shameful nor disloyal to recognize the point when a change needs to be made, and act accordingly. This may mean that placement in a facility needs to occur. Or it may mean that another family member needs to take over the task of caring for the loved one at home. It is wise for care partners to develop a plan, well before it becomes necessary, regarding what they will do if they are no longer able to continue providing care. Having to make these arrangements in haste (if, for example, the primary family care partner were to become acutely ill) is always more difficult and often results in a less satisfactory solution. Visiting local care facilities and discussing with other family members or a financial adviser the economic requirements ahead of time will make the task much easier when the time comes. But the greatest obstacle to overcome is often the attitude of the family care partner, who strongly resists considering that institutional placement may ever be necessary or even acceptable. Every family care partner should seriously consider how she will know when placement is inevitable and what steps she will take when that time comes. Making such preparations should, in fact, be viewed as an act of great loyalty and love.

Seeking Professional Help

When is it appropriate for the distressed care partner to seek professional help? There is no simple answer to that question, but it should be emphasized that, when in doubt, it is always better to seek counsel, whether from one's primary care physician, a member of the clergy, or a therapist, than to try to cope with significant distress alone. However, there are a number of objective signs that would call for the primary care partner to seek outside assistance. One sign would be that the care partner's life is being significantly and adversely affected by the tasks of providing care: for example, concentration, sleep, pleasure, or functioning on the job or at home with family are affected, or mood is significantly depressed. Of course, nearly every family care partner's life is adversely affected by being a care partner, so it is a matter of degree, and a judgment the care partner needs to make. Recognition of the need for help may not initially come from the care partner herself, but from friends or family who have noted that she is having a particularly difficult time. However, getting the family care partner to seek help may be a difficult task because of the stigma that so many feel about admitting a need and asking for help.

Another situation that calls for professional help is if the care partner finds himself becoming impatient or excessively irritated by the person with Alzheimer's. As noted before, every care partner feels irritation or impatience from time to time. It is, again, a matter of degree. As before, the primary care partner herself may not recognize or acknowledge the problem initially, but by good fortune, a friend or family member who is observing the situation will do so.

How does one begin to obtain help? For most family care partners, starting with the primary physician or care provider, or the physician who is treating the person with Alzheimer's disease is appropriate. Depending on the situation, the doctor treating the person with the disease may not be the best person to treat the care partner, as well. The care partner's own physician can examine the care partner for potential medical effects of stress (for example, elevated blood pressure) and may be able to directly address the concerns of the care partner. The primary physician can decide if a counselor is appropriate, if medication is warranted, or if a psychiatrist is needed in order to manage a more complex situation. The primary care provider may also refer the care partner to the Alzheimer's Association. Most chapters of the association have staff members who are expert in dealing with the typical challenges that arise for care partners, and they provide their services at no cost. On the other hand, a more complex or extensive issue may warrant a referral to a counselor or psychotherapist (the term, *therapist* is used to describe both counselors and psychotherapists here).

Whether the therapist is a social worker, a psychologist, a nurse practitioner, a pastoral counselor, or member of another discipline is generally less critical than whether or not the professional has experience in working with Alzheimer's care partners. A very good therapist with no experience in this area could be very helpful, but the challenges that arise in the life of someone who is a family care partner are unique and are best handled by someone who has specific experience in this area.

What can a therapist do? The distressed care partner may be aware of the need for some help (or may be led to it by concerned family or friends), but she may be unable to identify exactly why she is having so much difficulty, emotionally, with the task. It is the job of the therapist (with the help of the care partner) to identify what the difficulties are and to address them. Sometimes, simply having the opportunity to vent one's feelings about the situation is all that is necessary to help the stressed care partner. This is particularly true for the care partner who does not feel comfortable going to a support group. Ventilating ones feelings and concerns to a therapist can also give the care partner a feeling of "permission" to experience certain difficult emotions, as can also happen in a support group. Often, the experienced therapist is able to reassure the family care partner that her emotions are common ones felt by many care partners. When the therapist is able to suggest some useful methods for coping with such feelings, this can be most helpful.

At times, the care partner may feel particularly stressed by having to deal with difficult behavioral symptoms that the person with Alzheimer's is experiencing. Reading in books or attending lectures about how to handle such symptoms can be useful, but behavioral management advice regarding the specific details of the afflicted person's conduct from a therapist who also understands the care partner's particular personality and vulnerabilities can be invaluable.

In chapter 2, the various defenses that care partners use in an attempt to cope with the illness were considered. In most cases, the passage of time and the realities of the illness, along with the care partner's own emotional resilience will cause unhelpful defenses to give way to a more realistic view of the illness, even though that usually leads to more acute feelings of grief, as described. Sometimes, however, for a variety of reasons, family care partners are unable to move past the defenses they have employed to cope with the illness, and as a result, their understanding of and attitudes toward the disease and its management remain incomplete and unrealistic. This almost always leads to a great deal of stress, and it is unhealthy for both the care partner and the person with the disease. In this situation, a skillful therapist can help the care partner work through these defenses in a way that will allow her to proceed through the normal phases of grief, adaptation, and acceptance.

Just as some care partners may be unable to resolve their defensive views of the disease, other care partners may be unable to move beyond one of the common emotional reactions discussed in chapter 3. A care partner who remains profoundly guilty, or angry, or anxious, or ashamed is suffering beyond the usual misery of having a loved one with Alzheimer's; and it is also likely that the person with the disease is suffering unnecessarily, as a result. A therapist can help identify the emotion or emotions that are predominant and that are keeping the care partner from moving forward more productively.

Still other care partners may move past the defenses and challenging emotions described in chapters 2 and 3, but they are unable to work through the anguish of grief, toward adaptation and acceptance. In these cases, a therapist may be an essential aid.

One would hope that the immediate and more distant family members of someone with Alzheimer's disease are united in their view of the illness and the needs of the person with the disease, and that they are supportive of the primary family care partner. However, this is not always the case, unfortunately. The family care partner may sometimes experience a great deal of conflict or criticism from other family members at a time when just the opposite is needed. Often, this has to do with unresolved family issues, although it is possible that significant conflict can occur in families who have previously been quite close. When serious family conflict complicates the care situation, it can be very useful to be able to discuss these matters with an objective outsider, such as a therapist.

Finally, an important role for the therapist is to monitor the overall mental well-being of the family care partner, to make certain that he does not fall into a state of suicidal despair, or become abusive or neglectful. The therapist will also look for signs and symptoms of care partner burnout and, it is hoped, address these before damage is done to either person.

Psychiatric Help

When are the particular skills of a psychiatrist needed, rather than a non-physician therapist or primary care provider? Again, that may not be something that the distressed care partner can readily identify. However, in general, a psychiatrist may be specifically needed when it is determined that medication is indicated for the particular problem. That might be medication for sleep, or to treat depression, or severe anxiety. It might be the primary care provider who requests the aid of a psychiatrist, or a therapist might recognize that, in addition to the treatment he or she is offering, medication therapy might be necessary for the care partner.

A psychiatrist's skills might also be needed for the care partner who appears to be having unusual, atypical, or psychotic reactions to the stresses of providing care, or when there has been a history in the care partner of significant mental or emotional difficulties. Again, it might not be the care partner who would be expected to be able to determine this. In general, the primary care provider or the therapist would recognize that a consultation and/or treatment with a psychiatrist is necessary. Finally, it may be that, in a given community, it is a psychiatrist who is most experienced in managing patients and families with Alzheimer's disease and therefore is best equipped to deal with the emotional challenges of providing care, whether or not medication is warranted.

Epilogue

Having a loved one with Alzheimer's disease is a deeply painful experience. The progression of the illness, from its earliest stages to the end, is a saga of loss unmatched by most any other event. However, it *is* possible for the family care partner to survive the illness, emotionally. Ideally, she can reach a point of being capable of bidding farewell to her loved one, certainly with great sadness, but without bitterness. By the end of the journey, she can feel that she has gained something meaningful from the experience. She will feel ready and able to move forward with life after Alzheimer's. That this can happen is certainly a testament to human resilience and to the healing power of a loving relationship. But completing this journey successfully and with a measure of emotional equanimity is not easy.

It is hoped that the material presented in this volume has provided some valuable guidance toward this end, making it less arduous to cope with the many painful feelings along the way. The various emotional and psychological reactions of family care partners, from the earliest symptoms of the illness to the late stages of the disease, have been discussed in depth. As noted, these reactions do not occur in an organized, sequential fashion. Thus, while a family care partner may be attempting to deal with the discordance between herself and her loved one with regard to the severity or even the presence of the illness, she may at the same time be utilizing her own defenses to try to soften the blow of the awareness of certain especially painful elements of the disease. Simultaneously, she may be experiencing one or more intense emotions, such as guilt, anger, anxiety, or shame. And she may also be feeling a deep sense of loss and grief because of her awareness of the dire nature of the state of affairs.

That all of these different reactions and emotions happen concurrently, or in close proximity to one another, creates a very confusing and at times overwhelming situation, indeed. But the care partner's reactions and emotions are brought about by various factors, including her own personality, the nature and quality of her relationship with the afflicted individual, current symptoms of the illness, and present life events, to name a few.

One of the important tasks the family care partner must undertake is to address the basic differences between her views of the illness and those of the person with Alzheimer's disease. It is hard to move forward emotionally with the process of coping when there is a basic disagreement as to the nature or extent of the problem, or if, indeed, a problem even exists. This discordance can be a significant source of tension. While it is usually noted very early in the disease process, there may be some degree of discordance throughout the illness. Anosognosia, one important element of discordance, tends to increase as dementia worsens, although that does not automatically mean that discordance increases over time—other factors, including the efforts of the care partner, and the frequent confrontations with reality that occur as the disease worsens, may cause discordance to actually lessen over time. However, as new symptoms of the illness appear or new stages of impairment are reached, discordance can again become pronounced at any stage in the process. In some situations, it is present throughout the course of the illness and adds immeasurably to the stress of coping with it.

Both the care partner and the afflicted individual will cope much better with the illness, overall, if the basic issue of discordance is addressed. Alzheimer's disease is a major, life-altering phenomenon for the entire family, and it is critical that there be some common ground for discussion between the individual with the disease and his family members. At the outset, it may seem impossible to achieve this, but in most cases, that is not the case. Reducing discordance so that there is an opportunity for dialogue may require a number of very difficult discussions, but it is very much worth the effort involved.

The care partner's defenses were discussed in chapter 2. It is not possible, nor would it even be desirable, to eliminate all of the care partner's defenses against her full awareness of the disease, and all of its implications. This would be unbearably painful and frightening. Defenses serve an important function for everyone. In the care partner's case, they permit her to face the very unpleasant realities of the disease—and the grief that is at the center of her reaction to it—in a more gradual fashion, rather than overwhelming her all at once. In some cases, however, instead of allowing a gradual awareness of the painful realities of the situation, excessive or very rigid use of defenses can interfere with the care partner's coming to terms with the illness, and with her own grief. Having a solid understanding of the role that defenses play in the family care partner's psyche, combined with a great deal of honest self-reflection and insight, may make it possible for the family care partner to recognize when she is acting overly defensively and to modify this, in the direction of a more reality-based view of the current state of affairs.

Nearly every family care partner will experience at least one of the common emotional reactions presented in chapter 3. It can be helpful to know that these are indeed common reactions among care partners and to understand them in depth. Some family care partners are flooded with significant anxiety at certain stages of the illness, or throughout the entire course of the illness. Others find themselves feeling guilty that they are not doing enough for the person with Alzheimer's or that their relationship with the loved one over the years has somehow contributed to the development the disease. Another common guilt response is that she, the care partner, should not be permitted to enjoy her life in any way, because of the loved one's predicament. Still others find themselves feeling angry much of the time and drawing away from the person with the disease—when just the opposite is what is needed. These angry feelings can lead to significant guilt, as well, as the care partner knows, on some level, that the afflicted person is not able to control those behaviors that are provoking such ire. And there are some family care partners who feel very ashamed by the illness and by the behavior of the person afflicted.

Not only are these feelings painful to experience, particularly when they are very prominent, but they can interfere with the care partner's experiencing the grief that is at the center of her journey. In this way, these emotions can act like defense mechanisms. Of course, they are very genuine emotions, brought about by the loved one's illness, and in the context of the family care partner's personality and other factors. But to the extent that the care partner is preoccupied with one of these emotions—guilt, anger, anxiety, or shame—she cannot completely experience the sense of loss and grief that lie at the core of her emotional reaction to having a loved one with Alzheimer's disease.

How is this loss and grief experienced? First, it does not follow neatly after the discordance, the defenses, and the four emotions discussed above have presented themselves. Grief is a pervasive factor that is felt to some extent throughout the process. But it is felt perhaps most intensely, and can most readily be worked through, after the family member has, at least to some extent, understood and resolved her own defenses and has come to terms with the emotional challenges discussed above.

There are three phases, or components, of grief: the *anguish* associated with first coming to terms with the painful feelings of loss created by the disease; then, the many *adaptations* that must be made in order to continue to relate to someone who is being lost to Alzheimer's; and finally, *acceptance*. Acceptance is so much more than a simple intellectual understanding of the nature of the disease; it is, rather, an emotional recognition that the person, and one's relationship with him, has forever changed. It is only when a level of acceptance has been reached that genuine healing and moving forward can take place.

Although much of the psychological journey of the Alzheimer's family is internal, there are critical components of this process that must occur in a social, interpersonal context. Because of the stigma and shame so often associated with Alzheimer's disease, the risks of suffering in silence, or in a state of "disenfranchised grief," is very real. The benefits that accrue to the Alzheimer's family member from sharing openly with others—especially, those in the Alzheimer's community who have had similar experiences and feelings—are invaluable, and absolutely essential to reach the degree of acceptance that will allow her to move beyond grief and forge a new identity after coping so long with the emotional burdens of this disease.

This journey is one of the most stressful any individual can undertake. Chapter 8 discusses some of the causes of stress, as well as the impact it can have on the care partner, and also on the person with the disease. It describes a number of tools that the family member can utilize to help her cope with the stress. Finally, a number of resources are discussed that one can utilize when it doesn't seem possible, or wise, to manage without external help.

References

Books and Articles

Adelman, R. D., Tmanova, L. L., Delgado, D., et al. (2014): Caregiver burden: A clinical review. *JAMA* 311(10): 1052–1060.

Alzheimer's Association (2014): *2014 Alzheimer's Disease Facts and Figures*. Chicago: Alzheimer's Association.

American Psychiatric Association (2013): *Diagnostic and Statistical Manual of Mental Disorders*. 5th ed. Arlington, VA: American Psychiatric Publishing.

Beatty, W. W., Winn, P., Adams, R. L., et al. (1994): Preserved cognitive skills in dementia of the Alzheimer's type. *Archives of Neurology* 51: 1040–1046.

Bell, V., and Troxel, D. (2012): *A Dignified Life, Revised and Expanded: The Best Friends Approach to Alzheimer's Care; A Guide for Caregivers*. Deerfield Beach, FL: Health Communications.

Boss, P. (1999): *Ambiguous Loss*. Cambridge, MA: Harvard University Press.

——— (2013): *Loving Someone Who Has Dementia: How to Find Hope While Coping with Stress and Grief*. San Francisco: Wiley.

Bowlby, J. (1980): *Attachment and Loss:* Volume 3, *Sadness and Depression*. New York: Basic Books.

Brackey, J. (2011): *Creating Moments of Joy for the Person with Dementia*. West Lafayette, IN: Purdue University Press.

Braff, S., and Olenik, M. R. (2002): *Staying Connected While Letting Go: The Paradox of Alzheimer's Caregiving*. New York: M. Evans and Co.

Bryant, R. A. (2013): Is pathological grief lasting more than 12 months grief or depression? *Current Opinion in Psychiatry* 26(4): 41–46.

Carpenter, B. D., Xiong, C., Porensky, E. K., et al. (2008): Reaction to a dementia diagnosis in individuals with Alzheimer's disease and mild cognitive impairment. *Journal of the American Geriatrics Society* 56(3): 405–412.

Cohen, C. A., et al. (2002): Positive aspects of caregiving: Rounding out the caregiver experience. *International Journal of Geriatric Psychiatry* 17: 184–188.

Contador, I., Fernandez-Calvo, B., Palenzuela, D. L., et al. (2012): Prediction of burden in family caregivers of patients with dementia: A perspective of optimism based on generalized expectancies of control. *Aging and Mental Health* 16(6): 675–682.

Cooper, C., Katona, C., Orrell, M., and Livingston, G. (2006): Coping strategies and anxiety in caregivers of people with Alzheimer's disease: The LASER-AD study. *Journal of Affective Disorders* 90(1): 15–20.

Dichter, G. S. (2010): Anhedonia in unipolar major depressive disorder: A review. *Open Psychiatry Journal* 4: 1–9.

Doka, K. J. (2002): *Disenfranchised Grief: New Directions, Challenges, and Strategies for Practice*. Champaign, IL: Research Press.

Fostino, M. (2007): *Alzheimer's: A Caretaker's Journal*. New York: Seaboard Press.

Fox, J. (2009): *I Still Do: Loving and Living with Alzheimer's*. New York: Powerhouse Books.

Frank, J. B. (2008): Evidence for grief as the major barrier faced by Alzheimer's caregivers: A qualitative analysis. *American Journal of Alzheimer's Disease and Other Dementias* 22(6): 516–527.

Freud, A. (1937): *The Ego and the Mechanisms of Defense*. London: Hogarth Press and Institute of Psycho-Analysis.

Freud, S. ([1917] 1956–1974): *Mourning and Melancholia*. In *The Standard Edition of the Complete Psychological Works of Sigmund Freud*, 14: 243–258. London: Hogarth Press.

Garand, L., Lingler, J. H., Deardorf, K. E., et al. (2012): Anticipatory grief in new family caregivers of persons with mild cognitive impairment and dementia. *Alzheimer Disease and Associated Disorders* 26(2): 159–165.

Glenner, J. A., Stehman, J. M., Davagning, J., et al. (2005): *When Your Loved One Has Dementia: A Simple Guide for Caregivers*. Baltimore: Johns Hopkins University Press.

Green, C. R., and Beloff, J. (2008): *Through the Seasons: An Activity Book for Memory-Challenged Adults and Care Partners*. Baltimore: Johns Hopkins University Press.

Gústafsdóttir, M. (2011): Beneficial care approaches in specialized daycare units for persons with dementia. *American Journal of Alzheimer's Disease and Other Dementias* 26(3): 240–246.

Jolley, D. J., and Benbow, S. M. (2000): Stigma and Alzheimer's disease:

Causes, consequences, and a constructive approach. *International Journal of Clinical Practice* 54(2):117–119.

Jones, G. M. M. (2012): *The Alzheimer Café: Why It Works*. Suninghill, UK: Wide Spectrum Publishing.

Kahn, P. V., Zimmerman, C. O., Wishart, H. A., Santulli, R. B., and Werner, P. (2014): Caregiver stigma and burden in Alzheimer's disease: A comparison of spousal and adult children caregivers. Poster presented at the American Association for Geriatric Psychiatry Annual Meeting, March.

Koenig-Coste, J. (2003): *Learning to Speak Alzheimer's*. New York: Houghton Mifflin.

Kuhn, D. (2013): *Alzheimer's Early Stages: First Steps for Family, Friends, and Caregivers*. 3rd ed. Alameda, CA: Hunter House.

Lee, S. M., Roen, K., and Thornton, A. (2014): The psychological impact of a diagnosis of Alzheimer's disease. *Dementia* 13(3): 289–305.

Lindemann, E. (1944): The symptomatology and management of acute grief. *American Journal of Psychiatry* 101: 141–148.

Loi, S. M., Dow, B., Ames, D., et al. (2014): Physical activity in caregivers: What are the psychological benefits? *Archives of Gerontology and Geriatrics* 59(2): 204–210.

Mace, N. L., and Rabins, P. V. (2012): *The Thirty-Six Hour Day: A Family Guide to Caring for Persons with Alzheimer's Disease, Related Dementias Illnesses, and Memory Loss*. 5th ed. Baltimore: Johns Hopkins University Press.

Marist Institute for Public Opinion (2012): Alzheimer's most feared disease. Poll released November 14. http://maristpoll.marist.edu/1114-alzheimers-most-feared-disease, accessed June 15, 2014.

Martin, Y., Gilbert, P., McEwan, K., and Irons, C. (2006): The relation of entrapment, shame and guilt to depression, in carers of people with dementia. *Aging and Mental Health* 10(2): 101–106.

Mayo Clinic (2009): *Mayo Clinic Guide to Alzheimer's Disease*. Rochester, MN: Mayo Clinic.

McCurry, S. M., Logsdon, R. G., Teri, L., and Vitiello, M. V. (2007): Sleep disturbances in caregivers of persons with dementia: Contributing factors and treatment implications. *Sleep Medicine Reviews* 11(2): 143–153.

McLaughlin, M. (2013): Zen and the art of Alzheimer's. *Huffington Post*,

December 9. http://www.huffingtonpost.com/mary-mclaughlin/coping-with-alzheimers-_b_4405798.html.

Mittelman, M. S., Ferris, S. H., Shulman, E., Steinberg, G., and Levin, B. (1996): A family intervention to delay nursing home placement of patients with Alzheimer disease: A randomized controlled trial. *JAMA* 276(21): 1725–1731.

Normann, H. K., Norberg, A., and Asplund, K. (2002): Confirmation and lucidity during conversations with a woman with severe dementia. *Journal of Advanced Nursing* 39(4): 370–376.

Noyes, B. B., Hill, R. D., Hicken, B. L., et al. (2010): The role of grief in dementia caregiving. *American Journal of Alzheimer's Disease and Other Dementias* 25(1): 9–17.

Ogden, S. K., and Biebers, A. D. (2010): *Psychology of Denial*. Psychology of Emotions, Motivations and Actions Series. Hauppauge, NY: Nova Science Publishers.

Oken, B. S., Fonareva, I., Haas, M., et al. (2010): Pilot Controlled Trial of Mindfulness Meditation and Education for Dementia Caregivers. *Journal of Alternative and Complementary Medicine* 16(10): 1031–1038.

Ott, C. H., Sanders, S., and Kelber, S. T. (2007): Grief and personal growth experience of spouses and adult-child caregivers of individuals with Alzheimer's disease and related dementias. *Gerontologist* 47(6): 798–809.

Quinn, C., Clare, L., and Woods, R. T. (2012): What predicts whether caregivers of people with dementia find meaning in their role? *International Journal of Geriatric Psychiatry* 27(11): 1195–1202.

Richardson, T. J., Lee, S. J., Berg-Weger, M., and Grossberg, G. T. (2013): Caregiver health: Health of caregivers of Alzheimer's and other dementia patients. *Current Psychiatry Reports* 15(7): 367.

Rubinstein, N. (2011): *Alzheimer's Disease and Other Dementias: The Caregiver's Complete Survival Guide*. Minneapolis: Two Harbors Press.

Sanders, S., Ott, C. H., Kelber, S. T., and Noonan, P. (2008): The experience of high levels of grief in caregivers of persons with Alzheimer's disease and related dementia. *Death Studies* 32(6): 495–523.

Santulli, R. B. (2011): *The Alzheimer's Family: Helping Caregivers Cope*. New York: W.W. Norton.

——, ed. (2013): *The Dartmouth Memory Handbook*. 4th ed. Hanover, NH: Hanover Printing.

Schultz, R., and Martire, L. M. (2004): Family caregiving of persons with dementia: Prevalence, health effects and support strategies. *American Journal of Geriatric Psychiatry* 12(3): 240–249.

Schultz, R., Boerner, K., Shear, K., et al. (2006): Predictors of complicated grief among dementia caregivers: A prospective study of bereavement. *American Journal of Geriatric Psychiatry* 14(8): 650–658.

Schultz, R., Herbert, R., and Boerner, K. (2008): Bereavement after caregiving. *Geriatrics* 63(1): 20–22.

Semiatin, A. M., and O'Connor, M. K. (2012): The relationship between self-efficacy and positive aspects of caregiving in Alzheimer's disease caregivers. *Aging and Mental Health* 16(6): 683–688.

Sifton, E. (2003): *The Serenity Prayer: Faith and Politics in Times of Peace and War.* New York: W.W. Norton.

Starkstein, S. E., Jorge, R., Mizrahi, R., and Robinson, R. G. (2006): A diagnostic formulation for anosognosia in Alzheimer's disease. *Journal of Neurology, Neurosurgery and Psychiatry* 77(6): 719–725.

Tabak, N., Ehrenfeld, M., and Alpert, R. (1997): Feelings of anger among caregivers of patients with Alzheimer's disease. *International Journal of Nursing Practice* 3(2): 84–88.

Takai, M., Takahashi, M., Iwamitsu, Y., et al. (2009): The experience of burnout among home caregivers of patients with dementia: Relations to depression and quality of life. *Archives of Gerontology and Geriatrics* 49(1): e1–e5.

Vaillant, G. E. (1992): *Ego Mechanisms of Defense: A Guide for Clinicians and Researchers.* Washington, DC: American Psychiatric Publishing.

Wayman, L. (2011): *A Loving Approach to Dementia Care: Making Meaningful Connections with the Person Who Has Alzheimer's Disease.* Baltimore: Johns Hopkins University Press.

Werner, P., and Heinik, J. (2008): Stigma by association and Alzheimer's disease. *Aging and Mental Health* 12(1): 92–99.

Werner, P., Mittelman, M. S., Goldstein, D., and Heinik, J. (2012): Family stigma and caregiver burden in Alzheimer's disease. *Gerontologist* 52(1): 89–97.

Whitebird, R. R., Kreitzer, M. J., Crain, A. L., et al. (2013): Mindfulness-based stress reduction for family caregivers: A randomized controlled trial. *Gerontologist* 53(4): 676–686.

Yale, R. (1995): *Developing Support Groups for Individuals with Early-*

Stage Alzheimer's Disease: Planning, Implementation, and Evaluation. Baltimore: Health Professions Press.

Zarit, S. H. (2012): Positive aspects of caregiving: More than looking on the bright side. *Aging and Mental Health* 16(6): 673–674.

Useful Websites

The Alzheimer's Association
http://www.alz.org

Alzheimer's Foundation of America (AFA)
http://www.alzfdn.org

Caregiver Action Network
http://caregiveraction.org

Caring.com
http://www.caring.com

Caring from a Distance
http://www.cfad.org

Family Caregiver Alliance
http://www.caregiver.org

Helpguide.org
http://www.helpguide.org

MedlinePlus Health Information on Alzheimer's Disease
http://www.nlm.nih.gov/medlineplus/alzheimersdisease.html

National Alliance for Caregiving
http://www.caregiving.org

The National Institute on Aging Alzheimer's Disease Education and Referral Center
http://www.alzheimers.org/index.html

Index